Career Paths in Forensic Psychology

Career Paths in Forensic Psychology offers a comprehensive introduction and guide to the varied career paths for aspiring forensic psychologists, showing what a rewarding career at the intersection of law and psychology can look like in practice.

The book is divided into five parts. Part I provides an overview of the field of forensic psychology and also briefly explores its origins and evolution in the United States. Additionally, it explores common professional activities of forensic psychologists, as well as common career settings in which they ply their trade (academic settings, clinical settings, policy settings). Part II examines employment in academic settings, chiefly research academia, practice-oriented academia, and teaching-focused academia. Part III discusses opportunities for clinical-forensic psychology practice, in both the public sector and in private practice settings. Part IV considers career opportunities for policy-interested forensic psychologists, including in government agencies and policy-focused non-profit organizations. Finally, Part V gives readers tips on how to pick the best career "home base" for themselves, considers supplemental opportunities that forensic psychologists can pursue if their "home base" does not scratch all their professional itches, and provides guidance on how to put one's best foot forward as a forensic psychologist and be a worthy representative of the field.

This book is an ideal resource for students of forensic psychology and early-career forensic psychologists looking to start and progress their career in academic, clinical, and policy settings, as well as practicing psychologists looking to navigate career changes and transitions.

Jaymes Fairfax-Columbo, J.D., Ph.D., is a forensic mental health policy professional at a non-profit organization on the East Coast, U.S.A. He also maintains a forensic mental health evaluation and consulting private practice. Additionally, he is Visiting Assistant Professor of Psychology at Drexel University's Department of Psychological and Brain Sciences in Philadelphia, Pennsylvania, U.S.A. His research interests include mental health policy, forensic mental health assessment, therapeutic jurisprudence, and the prevention and reduction of criminal behavior and recidivism.

Alisha Desai, Ph.D., is a licensed clinical psychologist and founder of the Center for Values-Based Living, a mental health private practice and consulting firm. Her research and clinical interests focus on trauma, burnout, and compassion fatigue across the healthcare, humanitarian aid, and criminal legal sectors.

Simone Grisamore, M.S., is a doctoral student in the clinical psychology Ph.D. program at Drexel University in Philadelphia, Pennsylvania, U.S.A. Her research and clinical interests include community-based alternatives to incarceration and the treatment of mental health and substance use disorders.

David DeMatteo, J.D., Ph.D., ABPP (Forensic), is Professor of Psychology and Professor of Law at Drexel University in Philadelphia, Pennsylvania, U.S.A., and Director of Drexel's J.D./Ph.D. Program in Law and Psychology. He is Fellow of the American Psychological Association (Divisions 1, 12, and 41) and is board-certified in forensic psychology by the American Board of Professional Psychology. He is a former president of the American Psychology-Law Society (Division 41 of the American Psychological Association) and the American Board of Forensic Psychology, and he is Editor-in-Chief of *Law and Human Behavior*.

Career Paths in Forensic Psychology

A Primer for a Rewarding Career at the Intersection of Law and Psychology

Jaymes Fairfax-Columbo,
Alisha Desai,
Simone Grisamore and
David DeMatteo

Routledge
Taylor & Francis Group

NEW YORK AND LONDON

Designed cover image: Getty Images @erhui1979

First published 2026
by Routledge
605 Third Avenue, New York, NY 10158

and by Routledge
4 Park Square, Milton Park, Abingdon, Oxon, OX14 4RN

Routledge is an imprint of the Taylor & Francis Group, an informa business

ISBN: 9781032528724 (hbk)
ISBN: 9781032519760 (pbk)
ISBN: 9781003408857 (ebk)

DOI: 10.4324/9781003408857

Typeset in Bembo
by Apex CoVantage, LLC

Contents

Preface

The rapid and substantial growth of the field of forensic psychology over the past several decades prompted three of the authors to write *Becoming a Forensic Psychologist*, published in 2020. Several years later, this rapid and substantial growth has not slowed down! Psychological expertise pertaining to legal contexts is still in extremely high demand. Further, contemporary issues regarding the overlap between mental health and law—such as the seeming criminalization of mental illness, the Opioid Epidemic, the so-called Competency Services Crisis, and others—have placed the field of forensic psychology firmly in view of both policymakers and the public. In short, demand for the knowledge, skillset, and services of forensic psychologists has never been higher.

Given this, it should come as no surprise that interest in forensic psychology as a profession has also grown significantly in recent decades. Forensic psychology training programs continue to emerge and proliferate and at multiple levels (undergraduate, graduate, pre-doctoral internship training, postdoctoral fellowships). One oft-neglected focus of training programs in forensic psychology, though, is answering a simple question for trainees: What are the varied career paths that forensic psychologists can travel down?

That question was the impetus for this book. The authors span multiple career stages: doctoral graduate student (Simone Grisamore), early-to-mid career professionals (Alisha Desai and Jaymes Fairfax-Columbo), and a well-established professional who has forgotten more about forensic psychology than most will ever learn (Dave DeMatteo). Collectively, we have also had experience in *every* professional setting that this book explores. Regardless of our career stage or our current professional setting, we all agree that many prospective—and practicing—forensic psychologists are woefully unaware of the sheer *breadth* of opportunities that exist to ply our trade.

This book focuses on helping prospective and practicing forensic psychologists to determine the ideal career "home base" for themselves. Simply put, a "home base" is your primary career setting—which does not mean it is your only career setting. The book also focuses more broadly on how forensic psychologists might self-actualize, both in terms of their professional lives and their personal lives.

Career Paths in Forensic Psychology: A Primer for a Rewarding Career at the Intersection of Law and Psychology is divided into five parts. Part I, *Laying the Foundation*, provides an overview of the field of forensic psychology (Chapter 1), the common professional activities of forensic psychologists (Chapter 2), and common settings in which forensic psychologists might work (Chapter 3). In Part II, *Not Just an Ivory Tower: An Exploration of Academic Opportunities in Forensic Psychology*, we explore career options in research academia (Ph.D. programs, Chapter 4); we also consider careers in practice-oriented academia (Psy.D. programs, academic health centers, law schools) and teaching-focused academia (Chapter 5).

Part III, *Working with Individuals: An Exploration of Clinically Focused Jobs*, explores public sector (Chapter 6) and private practice opportunities (Chapter 7) for clinical-forensic psychologists. In Part IV, *Accomplishing System-Level Change: An Exploration of Policy Work in Forensic Psychology*, we examine the two primary settings where forensic psychologists engage in policy work: within government agencies (Chapter 8) and as part of a non-profit agency (Chapter 9). Finally, in Part V, *Putting It All Together: An Exploration of How to Actualize Your Career in Forensic Psychology*, we offer tips for helping readers to select the most appropriate career "home base" for them (Chapter 10), to consider low-burden supplemental opportunities to help them round out their career if their "home base" does not scratch all of their professional itches (Chapter 11), and to put their best foot forward as a forensic psychologist and as a representative of our field (Chapter 12).

This book can be read in two ways. First, it can be read from cover to cover. This method is likely most appealing for prospective forensic psychologists who want a comprehensive overview of all the career options that are open to them. Second, each chapter can be read in standalone fashion. This is likely most helpful for practicing forensic psychologists who are curious about options outside of their current (or past) career "home base." Given this dual readership strategy, some information may be repeated in several chapters. However, given the unique focuses of each chapter—and because the chapters have different primary authors and voices—we expect that it does not feel repetitive, even if you find that some information is repeated.

In addition to merely providing information about various career paths, we also wanted to give readers a true sense of what these paths look like *when walked in practice*. To that end, chapters in Parts II, III, and IV feature one or two *Career Profiles*. These *Career Profiles* explore the current career setting the writer works in, what got them interested in their current career path, what an average workday looks like for them, what they feel is the most rewarding aspect of their work, and some of the challenges in their chosen career path. All *Career Profile* writers also offer readers some guidance and advice for how to follow in their footsteps, should readers so choose. A very special thanks to all our *Career Profile* writers: Natalie M. Anumba, Ph.D., ABPP (Forensic); Natalie Armstrong, Ph.D. ABPP (Forensic); Cassandra Bailey, Ph.D.; Stephanie Brooks Holliday, Ph.D.; Jennifer Cox, Ph.D.; Heath Hodges, Ph.D., M.L.S., ABPP (Forensic); Christopher King, J.D., Ph.D.; Anthony Perillo, Ph.D.; Mina Ratkalkar, Ph.D.; and Matthew Stimmel, Ph.D.

We hope that this book helps serve as a roadmap to a rich and fulfilling career as a forensic psychologist. We hope that it helps prospective and practicing forensic psychologists to consider the myriad ways and in the myriad settings that forensic psychology expertise is *extremely* valuable. We hope that this book helps fill in a training, mentorship, and professional development gap experienced by many in our field. We hope this book encourages readers not to feel locked-in to more traditional professional trajectories but helps them think more flexibly and creatively about how they can best achieve a rewarding career. Most importantly, we hope this book inspires readers to find the career "home base" that best helps them self-actualize as a forensic psychologist.

If you are a potential forensic psychologist, best of luck as you ponder the best career trajectory for you. If you are currently a practicing forensic psychologist, best of luck in taking a step back and engaging in a critical examination of what will help you feel most professionally fulfilled. Regardless of where you are in your professional journey, happy reading!

Jaymes Fairfax-Columbo
Alisha Desai
Simone Grisamore
David DeMatteo

Part I

Laying the Foundation

CHAPTER 1

So . . . What Is Forensic Psychology, Anyway?

So you want to be a forensic psychologist, huh? Does the following sound familiar? True crime podcasts serve as the soundtrack to your life, and you read every true crime book you can get your hands on. While others are keeping up with the Kardashians, you are keeping up with Albert Fish, John Wayne Gacy, Jeffrey Dahmer, Ed Gein, Ted Kaczynski, and numerous others. You know mob history like the back of your hand and have seen *The Godfather*, *Goodfellas*, and *The Departed* too many times to count. You have your theories on who Jack the Ripper is, and you never miss an episode of *Unsolved Mysteries*. You've binged *Mindhunter* several times. All that is left for you to do is achieve your dream of becoming a criminal profiler with the FBI. Getting advanced training in forensic psychology is the final step remaining in your quest.

If this sounds familiar, you are not alone. When many think of forensic psychology, they think of the earlier example. In fact, the idea that forensic psychology is about criminal profiling is a common misconception that has greatly contributed to the explosive growth of interest in the field in recent years (Clay, 2009; Huss, 2001; Ward, 2013). That is not to say that psychologists are never involved in criminal profiling. For example, investigative psychologists help bolster the scientific rigor of law enforcement profiling methods (Winerman, 2004). However, most of the study and practice of forensic psychology *does not consist of* criminal profiling. So what exactly does forensic psychology entail? How might you know if a career in forensic psychology is the path for you? Read on to find out!

FORENSIC PSYCHOLOGY: FOUNDATIONAL TERMS

In operationalizing the study and practice of "forensic psychology," it is helpful to understand what each word means in isolation. The word *forensic* refers to "an activity or profession [that] is related to the law or a legal process"

DOI: 10.4324/9781003408857-2

(DeMatteo et al., 2020, p. 4). In this sense, "forensic" is a broad term that modifies the word it precedes, indicating the subsequent word is associated with the law. Consider the profession of a forensic accountant. Generally speaking, an *accountant* is someone who keeps track of a business' financial transactions. Accountants help businesses track profits and losses, generate balance sheets, conduct financial analyses to help businesses make informed decisions and understand and plan operating costs, and prepare taxes (Iwuozor & Main, 2023). As applied to the law, however, *forensic* accountants use the general accounting skills described earlier for narrower purposes. These include investigating whether an entity is engaging in financial reporting misconduct (i.e., fraud), an action that can bring about severe civil and criminal penalties. Their responsibilities may also include activities in support of litigation, including valuation of businesses, divorce valuations, estimating loss of earnings and projecting loss of future earnings, and investigating embezzlement (Honigsberg, 2020).

Now, let's look at the term *psychology*. Per the American Psychological Association (APA), "Psychologists examine the relationships between brain function and behavior, and the environment and behavior, applying what they learn to illuminate our understanding and improve the world around us" (*Science of Psychology*, n.d.). In short, *psychology* is concerned with how and why behavior manifests, whether due to differences in brain functioning or due to environmental influences.

Taken together, *forensic psychology* concerns how and why behavior manifests in the context of the legal system and as applied to legal concepts. Broadly, then, the practice of *forensic psychology* represents "the application of the science and practice of psychology to questions and issues relating to the law and the legal system" (DeMatteo et al., 2020, p. 5).

"FORENSIC": AN OVERVIEW OF THE AMERICAN LEGAL SYSTEM[1]

As stated earlier, forensic *psychology* refers to the application of psychology *to the legal system and to legal concepts*. For purposes of this book, we focus on psychology's application to the American legal system. Therefore, it is helpful to understand how the United States' (U.S.) legal system works. Though commonly referred to as a "democracy," the United States is a *representative democracy* and a *federal republic*. In essence, this means that in the U.S., citizens elect the individuals who they want to represent them in the government, and governmental power is dispersed among several levels: local, state, and national. Central to the American system of government are three concepts: federalism, separation of powers, and checks and balances.

Federalism

Federalism refers to governmental systems that disperse power among multiple levels of government (Cornell Law School, n.d.). The U.S. employs a system of dual sovereignty in which power is shared between a national government—called the federal government—and the various state governments. State governments also disperse power, with much policy being made at the local or municipal level (e.g., city, town). In the U.S., federalism is hierarchical; when there are conflicts between the various levels of government, federal law trumps state law and state law trumps local law.

Separation of Powers

Separation of powers refers to the idea that there should be multiple branches of government, each with a specialized function. At both the national and state levels, the U.S. splits governmental power among the Legislative Branch, the Executive Branch, and Judicial Branch. Per Article I of the U.S. Constitution, the Legislative Branch—also called the legislature—is tasked with creating laws. National and state legislatures consist of two bodies: the House of Representatives and the Senate. For proposed legislation (i.e., bills) to become law (i.e., statutes), they must be adopted by both bodies in the legislature. Municipalities also have legislative bodies, typically called councils, and the legislative acts that they pass are referred to as ordinances. Note that because the U.S. employs hierarchical federalism, ordinances only impact citizens who live in a municipality; state laws impact all citizens within that state, regardless of municipality; and federal laws impact all citizens in the United States, regardless of which state they live in. Consistent with the U.S. being a representative democracy, the citizenry elect members of the legislative bodies.

Per Article II of the U.S. Constitution, the Executive Branch—meaning the President at the federal level—is tasked with executing and enforcing the laws adopted by the legislature. The President does this by consulting with their Cabinet, comprised of the Vice President and the heads of various specialized agencies that advise the President on a small subset of priority issues. Such issues include agriculture, commerce, defense, education, energy, health, homeland security, housing, conservation, justice, labor, foreign policy, transportation, economic matters, and veterans (The White House, n.d.). Notably, in seeking to enforce the law, executive branch agencies often adopt enabling regulations or rules that help implement laws. These regulations are referred to as *administrative law*. Keeping federalism in mind, a *governor* is the state-level executive, while the executive is a *mayor* at the municipal level.

Governors and mayors similarly employ advisors to help them implement state laws and local ordinances. Consistent with the U.S. being a representative democracy, the citizens also elect presidents, governors, and mayors.

EXECUTIVE BRANCH AGENCIES: EXAMPLES

- Department of Agriculture
- Department of Defense
- Department of Energy
- Department of Homeland Security
- Department of Justice
- Department of State
- Department of the Treasury
- Environmental Protection Agency
- Small Business Administration

Under Article III of the U.S. Constitution, the Judicial Branch (also called the judiciary) comprises courts tasked with interpreting laws' meanings, as well as applying the law to individual cases and circumstances. Court systems in the U.S. generally have three levels: local courts (i.e., federal districts and state counties), also known as trial courts; appellate courts; and high courts (e.g., Supreme Courts). Trial courts apply laws to individual cases, and holdings at the local level only impact citizens of that district or county. Appellate courts—which also include high courts—review decisions made by lower courts to determine if some type of error was made in terms of how a case was handled and decided. Appellate courts can review decisions of trial courts, and high courts can review decisions of both trial and lower appellate courts. In the American legal system, the process of becoming a judge is more nuanced than the process of becoming a legislator or an executive. At the federal level, the President nominates judges for the Supreme Court of the United States (SCOTUS), for courts of appeals, and for district courts; these nominees need to be confirmed by the Senate. At the state level, the selection of judges varies by jurisdiction. Some states allow judges to be appointed by a governor, whereas in other states, the citizenry elect judges (Berkson, 1980).

Checks and Balances

Checks and balances is the final essential concept to the American system of government. Checks and balances ensure that no branch of government predominates over the others and becomes too powerful. Salient examples include the ability of an executive to veto legislation, the ability of the legislature to impeach an executive and to approve individuals the executive nominates for appointed positions (e.g., cabinet positions, appellate judges), and the ability of the courts to overturn laws that they deem unconstitutional (*Marbury v. Madison*, 1803).

CASE LAW REVIEW

Marbury v. Madison (1803) *established judicial review*, or the power of United States courts to determine that a law violates the Constitution (and is, therefore, invalid).

Sources of Law

In the U.S., there are four primary sources of law: constitutions, statutes, case law, and regulations (i.e., administrative law). Constitutions contain guiding principles from which all other lawmaking should follow, place restrictions on governmental power, and define the rights of the citizenry. Delegates at constitutional conventions create constitutions; these constitutions are then voted on by the citizenry for them to be adopted. Once a constitution is adopted, it typically is not replaced; if changes are desired, a constitution is instead amended. As previously mentioned, statutes (and ordinances) emanate from legislative bodies.

Case law emanates from courts. Courts consistently interpret and clarify the meanings of laws, and those interpretations carry forward. Courts also interpret and clarify constitutions and help to operationalize the rights of the citizenry and define the specific instances in which those rights can be abridged. For example, in *Dusky v. United States* (1960), SCOTUS held that the right to due process of law (a Fifth Amendment right) included the right to a competency determination prior to proceeding to trial; further, SCOTUS set the standard for *how* competency is determined (i.e., defendants must have a factual and rational understanding of the proceedings against them and be able to consult with their lawyers rationally).

Finally, as aforementioned, administrative law emanates from the Executive Branch. Administrative agencies pass regulations designed to help implement laws. Regulations do not in and of themselves have the force of law; rather, they reflect an administrative agency's *interpretation* of a law so as to enforce that law.

Criminal Law and Civil Law

A final important point about the American court system is that law is generally split into two systems: the criminal legal system and the civil legal system. Criminal law forbids individuals from engaging in behaviors that can be harmful to others. Legislatures pass laws explicitly proscribing certain behaviors. Individuals found to have engaged in these behaviors are held accountable and may face penalties, such as fines, probation, restitution payments, community service, incarceration, or execution. Criminal acts typically fall into one of three categories: felonies (serious crimes), misdemeanors (less serious crimes), or summary violations (petty offenses typically punished by fines). Criminal law is generally the domain of the states, though the federal government regulates criminal behavior that impacts federal issues (e.g., a crime against a federal representative or a crime that might impact interstate commerce, such as drug trafficking). Criminal proceedings always position the government as prosecutor against an individual as defendant.

KIDS ARE DIFFERENT

The juvenile justice system bears similarity to the criminal justice system in terms of proscribing certain behaviors. However, while the criminal justice system focuses on *punishment* to prevent recurrence of antisocial behavior, the juvenile justice system focuses on *rehabilitation*. This distinction recognizes that juvenile offenders have different capacities from adult offenders and, as such, require a different approach to preventing recurrence of delinquent behavior.

In contrast to criminal law, civil law seeks to remedy disputes between private parties concerning noncriminal rights. Such rights might include property rights, familial rights, tort claims in which individuals are compensated for legal wrongs committed by others, contract disputes, and equity claims (courts ordering a party to engage in a specific action). Civil proceedings may also concern an individual's liberty rights. For example, civil commitment, Sexually Violent Predator commitment, and guardianship proceedings are all types of civil proceedings. Generally, the parties to a civil case are usually private citizens, private entities, or business entities, though civil suits can also include the government. In civil proceedings, the party bringing the civil action is referred to as a plaintiff, and the party being sued is the defendant.

Both criminal and civil proceedings have similar elements. Generally speaking, both involve an adjudicative process in which two sides place evidence in dispute in an attempt to prove to a factfinder that their side of the case is correct. Once a factfinder determines culpability, a penalty or remedy is ordered. However, criminal and civil proceedings also have some distinct elements. The burden of proof in criminal proceedings is generally higher; culpability needs to be determined beyond a reasonable double. In contrast, the burden of liability in a civil proceeding is generally a preponderance of the evidence (i.e., more likely than not), though the burden can be higher in some proceedings (e.g., the lowest standard jurisdictions can use for civil commitment is clear and convincing evidence). The penalty/remedy in criminal proceedings and civil proceedings are also distinct. Individuals who commit criminal wrongs are punished, typically via the penalties mentioned earlier. In contrast, individuals/entities that commit civil wrongs are usually either ordered to compensate the plaintiff or to undergo a certain course of action.

"PSYCHOLOGY": SUBFIELDS OF PSYCHOLOGY AND HOW THEY INTERACT WITH THE LEGAL SYSTEM

Now that you have a basic understanding of the American system of government and law, we can turn to how *psychology* applies to this system. As indicated earlier, this book construes *forensic psychology* broadly as "the application of the science and practice of psychology to questions and issues relating to the law and the legal system" (DeMatteo et al., 2020, p. 5). Given that the field of psychology has multiple subfields, we will review several examples of how professionals might apply these subfields to the American legal system.

Cognitive Psychology

According to the American Psychological Association, cognitive psychology is the study of "how people acquire, perceive, process, and store information" (*Cognitive Psychology Explores our Mental Processes*, n.d.). As applied to the legal system, cognitive-forensic psychologists explore how *mental processes* impact decision making and the legal system. Salient examples include exploring what contributes to errors in eyewitness identification and testimony, cognitive biases in the investigative process, cognitive biases in jury and judge decision making, and cognitive biases in reaching opinions in forensic mental health assessments.

FORENSIC (NOT SO) FUN FACT

Inaccurate eyewitness identification is one of the leading causes of wrongful conviction. Eyewitness memories may be influenced by information provided after the fact; further, eyewitnesses are often overconfident in how accurate their memories are (Wise et al., 2014).

Clinical Psychology

Clinical psychology concerns the study of psychopathology and the provision of mental health treatment (*Clinical Psychology*, n.d.). As applied to the legal system, clinical-forensic psychologists engage in both evaluation and treatment. Regarding evaluation, clinical-forensic psychologists explore how psychopathology impacts *functional legal capacities,* and they also assess other legally relevant constructs, such as violence and/or recidivism risk or the suffering of a psychological injury. They may be called upon to conduct evaluations and testify in myriad legal contexts, including adjudicative competence, mental state at the time of the offense, *Miranda* rights waiver, civil commitment, guardianship, sentencing, juvenile transfer, personal injury, child custody, parental capacity, and others. Concerning treatment, clinical-forensic psychologists may provide therapeutic intervention to help individuals regain adjudicative competence (alternatively called competence to stand trial or competence to proceed), reduce risk of criminal behavior, and successfully reintegrate back into the community upon release.

KNOW THE LINGO

"Functional legal capacities" refer to functional demands that are expected of individuals in a specific legal context. Such capacities vary according to the legal issues presented (Heilbrun et al., 2009).

Though neurocognitive and neurodevelopmental disorders fall within the purview of clinical psychology, specializing in this type of psychopathology can often be helpful in legal contexts. To this end, forensic neuropsychologists largely concern themselves with how brain functioning impacts legal questions. Increasingly, individuals with complex neuropsychological conditions present in courtrooms; cases which involve assessment of dementia, assessment of Intellectual Disability or autism spectrum disorder, considerations of Fetal Alcohol Syndrome, or traumatic brain injuries may be particularly appealing for forensic neuropsychologists.

Developmental Psychology

Developmental psychology concerns itself with how people grow and develop across the lifespan. As applied to the legal system, developmental-forensic psychologists explore how progression along the lifespan impacts various legal issues. Common examples include researching adolescent decision making as it pertains to risky behavior or examining differences in children's abilities to navigate the legal system as compared to adults. For example, research suggests that adolescents are more susceptible to peer influence than adults and are more likely to engage in risky behaviors as a result (e.g., Albert et al., 2013). Additionally, research suggests that children and adolescents are more susceptible to providing false confessions and subsequently being wrongfully convicted than are adults (e.g., Kassin, 2017).

FORENSIC FUN FACT

Developmental-forensic psychologists were integral in helping SCOTUS understand differences between adolescent versus adult offenders. Their contributions helped lead SCOTUS to decisions that abolished the death penalty (*Roper v. Simmons*, 2005) and sentences of mandatory life without parole (*Miller v. Alabama*, 2014) for juvenile homicide offenders.

Social Psychology

The subfield of social psychology centers on how social environments influence both individual and group behavior (*Social Psychology Studies Human Interactions*, n.d.). As applied to the law, social-forensic psychologists study topics such as jury and judge decision making; perceptions of the legal system (e.g., deterrence theory, procedural justice); negotiation and plea bargaining; addressing racial bias and discrimination in the legal system; reducing bias in investigative procedures, such as police lineups; exploring factors increasing the likelihood of false confessions; shooter bias (the tendency to make decisions to shoot more quickly when individuals are of a racial/ethnic minority group); detection of deception; perceptions of culpability; jury selection; and crime prevention, among others. In fact, several essays in Hugo Münsterberg's (1908) *On the Witness Stand: Essays on Psychology and Crime*—the work credited with starting the field of forensic psychology in the United States—concern topics spanning social psychology and the law.

> ## FORENSIC (NOT SO FUN) FACT
> Did you know that many factors influence judges' decision making, including factors that have nothing to do with the defendant or the case? For example, a study in Israel found that judges gave more lenient sentences after they recharged with a meal break (Danzinger et al., 2011).

A BRIEF HISTORY OF FORENSIC PSYCHOLOGY IN THE UNITED STATES

The great Maya Angelou famously noted, "You can't really know where you're going until you know where you have been." As mentioned, forensic psychology started to gain footing in the United States with the 1908 publication of Hugo Münsterberg's *On the Witness Stand: Essays on Psychology and Crime*. In *On the Witness Stand*, Münsterberg advocated that psychological science could be applied to enrich the legal system. Throughout his work, he highlighted the fallibility of human memory, discussed how deception might be detected, sounded the alarm on false confessions and suggestibility in court, and pushed for prevention of crime (i.e., first contact with the criminal justice system) instead of prevention of recidivism (i.e., perpetual contact with the criminal justice system).

Where Münsterberg cracked a door, William Marston pushed the door open. Marston—trained dually as a lawyer and a psychologist—was appointed to the faculty of American University as a professor of legal psychology in 1922. Marston's research and scholarly pursuits helped lead to the invention of the polygraph and helped shed light on jury decision making; further, he is considered one of the first psychologists to heavily consult with criminal justice professionals. By the 1930s, numerous scholarly articles on the intersection between law and psychology had been published, as well as the first legal psychology textbook. By the 1940s and 1950s, psychologists were testifying in court on a regular basis, suggesting that the field of psychology was beginning to be taken seriously by legal professionals. In fact, social psychology studies were highly influential in SCOTUS's decision that "separate but equal" laws were unconstitutional in 1954's *Brown v. Board of Education* (Bartol & Bartol, 2013).

The 1960s saw federal support for clinical psychologists' involvement in the courtroom, with the United States Court of Appeals for the District of Columbia Circuit's decision to allow psychologists to testify in cases where mental illness was in question *(Jenkins v. United States, 1962). Previously, this was considered squarely to be the domain of psychiatrists. In 1968, the federal government began funding research on antisocial behavior via the National Institute of Mental Health's Center for Studies of Crime and Delinquency. By 1969, the field of forensic psychology had enough momentum to warrant the establishment of the American Psychology-Law Society (AP-LS)* (Grisso, 2018). In 1980, the American Psychological Association approved the Division of Psychology and Law (APA Div. 41). By 1984, the Division of Psychology and Law and AP-LS merged, with AP-LS now serving as Division 41 of the American Psychological Association.

Today, the field of forensic psychology enjoys a firm foothold in the U.S. Numerous forensic psychology training programs exist, offering graduate training, pre-doctoral internships, and postdoctoral fellowships (see later chapters in this book). Numerous peer-reviewed publication outlets exist, such as *Law and Human Behavior, Behavioral Sciences and the Law,* and *Criminal Justice and Behavior.* Forensic psychologists are increasingly turned to for expert evaluation and testimony in United States courts. Further, as of 2001, the American Psychological Association had designated forensic psychology as a specialty area of psychology (DeMatteo et al., 2020).

FORENSIC FUN FACT

Forensic psychologists have also been invited onto some of the most popular podcasts in the United States, speaking to massive listenership bases on important topics. Recent examples include Dr. Nancy Panza being interviewed on the *Joe Rogan Experience* (Rogan, 2020) or Dr. Saul Kassin being interviewed on *Armchair Expert* (Shepard, 2022).

CHAPTER TAKEAWAYS

The field of forensic psychology is expansive. From nearly nonexistent in the U.S. in the early 1900s to being one of the fastest growing subfields of psychology since the early 2000s, forensic psychology has arrived on the scene. Broadly construed, forensic psychologists represent numerous subfields of psychology—including cognitive, clinical, developmental, and social—and all focus on applying knowledge from that subfield to the American legal system and to legal issues. Such issues span both criminal law and civil law, and the practice of forensic psychology is influenced by lawmaking from all branches and at all levels of government. Now that you know *what forensic psychology is,* you can turn your attention to another daunting question: What do I want to do in the field of forensic psychology? You may not yet have an answer to that question, or you may simply feel like your options are too many and it's difficult to narrow down a solid career path. No need to worry; we've got you covered. Keep reading!

NOTE

1 A comprehensive review of the American legal system is beyond the scope of this book. For an expanded review, readers are referred to Chapter 1 of this book's predecessor, *Becoming a Forensic Psychologist* (DeMatteo et al., 2020), or to Chapter 2 of *Psychological Evaluations for the Courts: A Handbook for Mental Health Professionals and Lawyers, Fourth Edition* (Melton et al., 2018).

REFERENCES

Albert, D., Chein, J., & Steinberg, L. (2013). Peer influences adolescent decision making. *Current Directions in Psychological Science*, *22*(2), 114–120. https://doi.org/10.1177/0963721412471347

Bartol, C. R., & Bartol, A. M. (2013). History of forensic psychology. In I. B. Weiner & R. K. Otto (Eds.), *The handbook of forensic psychology* (4th ed., pp. 3–29). Wiley.

Berkson, L. C. (1980). Judicial selection in the United States—A special report. *Judicature*, *64*(4), 176–193.

Brown v. Board of Education of Topeka, 347 U.S. 482 (1954).

Clay, R. A. (2009). Postgrad growth area: Forensic psychology. *gradPSYCH Magazine*, 7(4). https://www.apa.org/gradpsych/2009/11/postgrad

Clinical psychology. (n.d.). American Psychological Association. https://www.apa.org/ed/graduate/specialize/clinical

Cognitive psychology explores our mental processes. (n.d.). American Psychological Association. https://www.apa.org/education-career/guide/subfields/brain-science

Cornell Law School. (n.d.). *Federalism*. Legal Information Institute. https://www.law.cornell.edu/wex/federalism

Danzinger, S., Levav, J., & Avaniam-Pesso, L. (2011). Extraneous factors in judicial decisions. *PNAS*, *108*(17), 6889–6892. https://doi.org/10.1073/pnas.1018033108

DeMatteo, D., Fairfax-Columbo, J., & Desai, A. (2020). *Becoming a forensic psychologist*. Routledge.

Dusky v. United States, 362 U.S. 402 (1960).

The Executive Branch. (n.d.). The White House. https://www.whitehouse.gov/about-the-white-house/our-government/the-executive branch/#:~:text=The%20Cabinet%20is%20an%20 advisory,often%20the%20President's%20closest%20confidants.

Grisso, T. (2018). The evolution of psychology and law. In T. Grisso & S. L. Brodsky (Eds.), *The roots of modern psychology and law: A narrative history* (pp. 1–37). Oxford University Press.

Heilbrun, K., Grisso, T., & Goldstein, A. M. (2009). *Foundations of forensic mental health assessment*. Oxford University Press.

Honigsberg, C. (2020). Forensic accounting. *Annual Review of Law and Social Science*, *16*, 147–164. https://doi.org/10.1146/annurev-lawsocsci-020320-022159

Huss, M. T. (2001). What is forensic psychology? It's not Silence of the Lambs! *Eye on Psi Chi*, *5*(3). https://www.psichi.org/page/053EyeSpring01cHuss

Iwuozor, J., & Main, K. (2023, January 20). What is accounting? The basics of accounting. *Forbes Advisor*. https://www.forbes.com/advisor/business/what-is-accounting/#:~:text=Accounting%20is%20the%20process%20of,legal%20reasons%20and%20 tax%20purposes

Jenkins v. United States, 307 F. 2d 637 (D.C. Cir. 1962).

Kassin, S. M. (2017). False confessions. *Wiley Interdisciplinary Reviews: Cognitive Science*, *8*(6), e1439. https://doi.org/10.1002/wcs.1439

Marbury v. Madison, 5 U.S. 157 (1803).

Melton, G. B., Petrila, J., Poythress, N. G., Slobogin, C., Otto, R. K., Mossman, D., & Condie, L. O. (2018). *Psychological evaluations for the courts: A handbook for mental health professionals and lawyers* (4th ed.). The Guilford Press.

Münsterberg, H. (1908). *On the witness stand: Essays on psychology and crime.* McClure.

Rogan, J. (Host). (2020, July 29). Nancy Panza (No. 1517) [Audio podcast episode]. In *The Joe Rogan Experience.* Spotify. https://open.spotify.com/episode/01A5ICPmRS5e dQeMIB71wn

Science of psychology. (n.d.). American Psychological Association. https://www.apa.org/education-career/guide/science

Shepard, D. (Host). (2022, September 29). Saul Kassin (psychologist on false confessions) [Audio podcast episode]. In *Armchair Expert.* Spotify. https://open.spotify.com/episod e/4ub97z86YPLes2g5ddea36

Social psychology studies human interactions. (n.d.). American Psychological Association. https://www.apa.org/education-career/guide/subfields/social

Ward, J. T. (2013). What is forensic psychology? *Psychology Student Network, 1*(2). https://www.apa.org/ed/precollege/psn/2013/09/forensic-psychology

Winerman, L. (2004). Criminal profiling: The reality behind the myth. *Monitor on Psychology, 35*(7), 66. https://www.apa.org/monitor/julaug04/criminal

Wise, R. A., Sartori, G., Magnussen, S., & Safer, M. A. (2014). An examination of the causes and solutions to eyewitness error. *Frontiers in Psychiatry, 5*, 102. https://doi.org/10.3389/fpsyt.2014.00102

CHAPTER 2

Gotcha . . . So What Do Forensic Psychologists Actually Do, Then?

Now that you have a better understanding of forensic psychology, you may be curious about the specific roles and responsibilities of a forensic psychologist. The professional activities of forensic psychologists generally align with those of the broader field of psychology, as they draw upon the principles of human behavior to offer expertise in psychological research, clinical practice, policy, and consultation. Uniquely, forensic psychologists expand beyond this foundation and utilize their knowledge in these areas to address issues and questions relating to the law.

In this chapter, we will delve into the professional activities in which forensic psychologists engage. It will become evident throughout this book that forensic psychology encompasses a wide range of professional activities. The scope of the field extends across various legal and policy issues pertaining to diverse age groups, individuals with mental illness, and justice-involved individuals. Moreover, it encompasses the various stages of the civil and criminal justice process and spans the intercepts of the sequential intercept model (Munetz & Griffin, 2006), from crisis de-escalation to reentry (we will explore this in more detail later in this book). As a forensic psychologist, you will have the opportunity to specialize in a specific area, or you may develop multiple specializations. Throughout this chapter, consider which activities resonate with you and align with your career goals. In subsequent chapters, we will explore how these activities can be incorporated into different career settings.

CLINICAL PRACTICE

When people think of psychologists, clinical practice is often the first thing that comes to mind. This perception holds true within forensic psychology, where clinical activities play a prominent role, although the nature of

DOI: 10.4324/9781003408857-3

clinical-forensic practice differs in important respects from more traditional clinical practice. Many forensic psychologists receive training in clinical practice and acquire the credentials required to provide and oversee assessments and interventions. Forensic psychology encompasses a wide range of clinical services, which can differ in terms of setting and objectives.

Forensic Mental Health Assessment

One of the most common activities of a forensic psychologist is conducting forensic mental health assessments (FMHA). FMHA are evaluations designed to convey relevant clinical information to legal stakeholders. The ultimate goal of an FMHA is to aid in informed legal decision making. Depending on the referral source, stakeholders may include attorneys, judges, probation/parole officers, parole boards, insurance companies, or state boards of psychology. FMHA can occur in both criminal and civil legal contexts, as well as in administrative contexts. In terms of process, the forensic evaluator conducts interviews with the criminal defendant or civil litigant, obtains and reviews relevant collateral information (such as medical records, educational records, legal records, or interviews with individuals who know the examinee), observes behavior, and administers and interprets psychological testing. The culmination of this assessment process is a deliverable conveying the evaluator's method, the data considered, and their findings, which is then provided to the party that requested the evaluation, typically the attorney or court (DeMatteo et al., 2020; Heilbrun et al., 2014). Delivery may take several forms, including verbal consultation, a written report, or testimony (in court or in a deposition).

GENERAL FLOW OF A FORENSIC MENTAL HEALTH ASSESSMENT

1. Referral (generally, court-ordered or attorney-retained).
2. Clarification of referral question.
3. Data gathering (interviews, psychological testing, record review, collateral contacts).
4. Deliverable (e.g., consultation, letter, report).
5. Testimony (if requested).

In some ways, the skillset required for conducting clinical assessments and FMHA is similar, but the purpose of the evaluation fundamentally differs. A clinical assessment aims to inform a psychological treatment plan to address symptoms of mental illness or to diagnose a disorder. On the other hand, an FMHA focuses on addressing a specific legal question. An FMHA may also include treatment recommendations or diagnoses, but they are only included to the extent that they are relevant to the legal question being addressed (DeMatteo et al., 2020).

The distinct purpose of FMHA has several implications for the activities and role of a forensic psychologist. For instance, in a clinical assessment, the individual being evaluated is considered the client. However, in an FMHA, the client is the stakeholder who requested the evaluation (e.g., an attorney or a court). Consequently, it is the forensic evaluator's job to maintain a neutral and objective role, rather than being in alliance with the examinee or providing therapeutic care. Another notable difference from a clinical assessment is the importance of ensuring the validity of the information gathered. In legal cases, there may be incentives to distort the information provided during any activity that involves self-report (e.g., clinical interview, some psychological testing). To ensure the validity of the information, forensic evaluators employ various techniques, such as reviewing available records, interviewing third parties, and utilizing psychological testing that assesses for misrepresented symptoms or the possibility that information provided may be misleading (called assessment of "response style"). Another essential element of FMHA that differentiates it from clinical assessment is the possibility of providing expert testimony. Psychologists retained as expert witnesses provide testimony regarding psychological issues in legal or administrative proceedings. In the case of an FMHA, forensic psychologists can provide opinion testimony based on data gathered during an assessment (for a comprehensive review, see DeMatteo et al., 2020).

Across all the activities of a forensic psychologist, we firmly emphasize the importance of having relevant training and expertise, particularly when it comes to FMHA. A significant portion of a forensic psychologist's work in the context of evaluations involves engaging with the legal system. This may include conducting assessments in a secure facility, interacting with attorneys, and effectively communicating the assessment findings in depositions, hearings, and trials. Therefore, it is crucial for a forensic psychologist to possess a fundamental understanding of the relevant legal proceedings and standards to be a proficient evaluator. It is also essential for performing FMHA to know the valid and reliable principles and methodology in the field. Being up to date on best practices enables the evaluator to select and use appropriate assessment tools and to provide informative and comprehensive testimony. FMHA serve a wide range of purposes, and the necessary skillset and knowledge vary depending on the type of case (American Psychological Association [APA], 2013; Heilbrun et al., 2014).

Criminal FMHA

Within the criminal justice context, FMHA serves various purposes, including providing sentencing recommendations, assessing specific criminal competencies, evaluating risk of future offending, assisting in determining the appropriate jurisdiction of a case (transferring the case to or from the juvenile court), and assessing criminal responsibility (Heilbrun et al., 2009). Two common criminal FMHA contexts are described later.

The most frequently conducted evaluations by forensic psychologists are adjudicative competence evaluations, often alternatively referred to as competence to stand trial or competence to proceed evaluations (Melton et al., 2018). Forensic psychologists play a crucial role in assisting the court to determine if an individual meets the legal requirements to proceed with their case. Adjudicative competence evaluations aid the court in determining if the individual meets the legal definition of competence. As defined by the United States Supreme Court in *Dusky v. United States* (1960), an individual is competent if they have a factual and rational understanding of the proceedings against them and the ability to assist counsel in their defense. Though *Dusky* controls only at the federal level, most states have adopted either the *Dusky* standard or a similar standard in terms of operationalizing adjudicative competency evaluations. When adjudicative competence becomes a concern—generally, due to being raised by the defense or the prosecution or raised *sua sponte* by a judge—an adjudicative competence evaluation is ordered. It then becomes the responsibility of the forensic evaluator to gather and present relevant data pertaining to the individual's competence to proceed and present this information to the court (Zapf & Roesch, 2009).

In both criminal (e.g., sentencing) and civil (e.g., Sexually Violent Predator) contexts, risk assessments are common. Risk assessments generally have the purpose of estimating an individual's likelihood of future antisocial behavior (e.g., violence, general recidivism, sexual recidivism), conceptualizing an individual's risk, and identifying ways to potentially mitigate that risk. These assessments can be applied to various legal questions, covering three primary areas: sentencing, supervised release, and the appropriate level of treatment based on the assessed risk (Monahan & Skeem, 2016). Forensic psychologists play a crucial role in risk assessment, which involves developing and validating instruments in research settings, selecting appropriate tools for assessment, administering and scoring assessments, and writing reports.

Civil FMHA

In the civil context, FMHA help address legal questions regarding issues that arise between two parties, including civil commitment, child custody, guardianship/conservatorship, employment discrimination or harassment, and psychological damages in personal injury cases (Heilbrun et al., 2009). Several common types of civil law FMHA are described later.

FMHA for psychological injuries are conducted in civil cases where an individual has sustained mental distress because of a threat or injury. Cases involving psychological injury encompass a wide range of legal questions, including those related to sexual harassment, workplace discrimination, medical malpractice, and police brutality. In these cases, the psychologist's role is to assess any emotional, psychological, or cognitive harms sustained by the injured party and to determine if the harm resulted from the behaviors of the defendant. The process for conducting an FMHA in the context of psychological injury shares similarities with that of criminal cases. An attorney or court typically requests the evaluation, and the psychologist's role is to address the specific legal question. The evaluation is centered around the legal question, and it is the role of the evaluator to filter through the information to determine what is relevant. This is typically accomplished by reviewing records, administering psychological testing, and conducting a clinical interview. Subsequently, the evaluator prepares a detailed report and may testify (Kane & Dvoskin, 2011).

In family law proceedings relating to child custody, FMHA evaluations can aid the court in a dispute over decision making, caretaking, and parental rights. The purpose of a child custody FMHA is to help the court render a decision regarding the children's best interests in a custody matter. The evaluation spans areas pertaining to a child's psychological interests and welfare, including factors related to psychological functioning, parenting, social, education, development, and the child's wishes. Efforts are made to examine all relevant parties, typically including both parents and children to determine the fit between parenting abilities and the children's needs. Other relevant data are also gathered, including psychological testing and information from schools, healthcare providers, childcare providers, family, and friends. The psychologist then conveys relevant findings to the courts (APA, 2022).

Administrative FMHA

Forensic psychologists may also conduct FMHA related to administrative questions. These evaluations occur within an office of the Executive Branch, compared to civil or criminal FMHA that occur in the Judicial Branch. Administrative evaluations may be used for occupational purposes, such as fitness to serve, licensure/certification, hiring decisions, and disability determinations. Police officers and public safety officials are often subject to these evaluations to determine if an individual meets specific guidelines for psychological suitability mandated by statutes, regulations, and policies (APA, 2018).

FORENSIC FUN FACT

More than 90% of state and local law enforcement require a psychological evaluation in the selection and hiring process (Reeves, 2012).

Forensic Treatment

Clinical-forensic psychologists can offer both forensic treatment and more generalized clinical treatment. It is important to note that just because a therapeutic service is provided to someone with justice involvement or is ordered by a court, that does not mean the provided treatment is forensic treatment (APA, 2013). Rather, forensic treatment is related to a specific psycholegal issue. For example, forensic psychologists may provide competency restoration treatment to defendants found incompetent to proceed. However, forensic psychologists can also provide more generalized clinical treatment to justice-involved populations. Examples might include delivering therapy for individuals with serious mental illnesses in state hospital or carceral settings (Huss, 2014). It can also include providing therapeutic services to help mitigate an offender's risk of recidivism. Again, the term *forensic* is broadly construed—if it involves or stems from the legal system, it is considered "forensic" for purposes of this book.

The content of the therapeutic services delivered can vary significantly based on the context of the situation. To illustrate, treatment within a carceral facility may look quite different from a community-based intervention, and the treatment for an individual convicted of one type of offense (e.g., a substance-related offense) may vary significantly from other offenses (e.g., sex offenses, violent offenses). This approach is not dissimilar from general clinical psychology practice in which individual needs and goals play a role in determining the course of treatment. In all these cases, a forensic psychologist providing clinical treatment may directly deliver services, oversee other clinical treatment staff, and/or assess the appropriateness of the treatment for the individual. Several examples of common types of treatment services that forensic psychologists might provide are reviewed later.

Competency Restoration

Individuals determined not competent to stand trial have a legal right to be restored to competency in the foreseeable future (*Jackson v. Indiana*, 1972). Many states have treatment programs to restore individuals to competence so the legal process can be resumed. Restoration treatment is ordered by courts and is most commonly delivered in a state hospital, but it can also be delivered in jails or the community. Treatment components typically include medication management, case management, and intervention focused on competence-related abilities (Heilbrun et al., 2019). The role of the forensic psychologist is to work in conjunction with a broader multidisciplinary team to deliver treatment and assess progress. A psychologist may deliver clinical treatment interventions, conduct assessments to determine progress and appropriate level of care, and serve as a liaison between the treatment facility and the courts.

FORENSIC FUN FACT

Evidence-based clinical treatments have also been adapted for potential utilization as an adjunctive treatment in competency restoration. For example, cognitive behavioral therapy for psychosis (CBT-p) focuses on reducing distress and improving quality of life while incorporating specific techniques to address psychotic symptoms. CBT-p may help curtail symptoms that may hinder an individual's participation in the legal process (Grossi et al., 2021).

Offender Rehabilitation

Various treatment modalities focus on rehabilitating offenders and reducing the probability of recidivism. Specific treatment approaches may be tailored to address unique characteristics based on the type of offense, such as a violent or sexual offense (Craig et al., 2013). For example, cognitive-behavioral therapy and relapse prevention therapy with a focus on regulating behavior and recognizing risks have demonstrated effectiveness in reducing risk of sexual recidivism (Kim et al., 2016). In addition to providing treatment, forensic psychologists may also conduct assessments before and after treatment, adapt and develop interventions for specific treatment needs, and coordinate treatment with the courts.

Offender rehabilitation efforts are often grounded in the risk-need-responsivity model (Bonta & Andrews, 2023). The framework encompasses three essential components for delivering effective intervention. The first principle is "risk," which involves identifying an individual's level of risk pertaining to future criminal offending. The intensity of any intervention provided should match the true level of risk an offender presents with; otherwise, the intervention may have iatrogenic effects (meaning it may make it more likely that the offender will recidivate). The second component of the model is the "need" principle. Criminogenic needs refer to risk factors that are associated with criminal offending and are modifiable via treatment. Examples include having a substance use disorder, holding pro-criminal attitudes, or frequently associating with antisocial peers. The third component, "responsivity," emphasizes tailoring treatment to the individual's unique characteristics. Recognizing that each person has distinct attributes or circumstances, interventions can be customized to align with their abilities, motivations, cultural backgrounds, and personal circumstances (e.g., having a serious mental illness that needs to be addressed, having an unstable housing or financial situation, etc.). This approach optimizes the effectiveness of treatment interventions, particularly for individuals involved with the justice system (Bonta & Andrews, 2023).

KNOW THE LINGO

Per the risk-need-responsivity model, there are eight key domains into which risk factors for generalized recidivism fall. These are [1] criminal history, [2] education/employment, [3] family/marital, [4] leisure/recreation, [5] companions, [6] alcohol/drug problem, [7] procriminal attitude/orientation, and [8] antisocial pattern.

RESEARCH

FORENSIC FUN FACT

Research indicates cognitive-behavioral programs that utilize a risk-need-responsivity approach result in substantial reductions in recidivism (Lipsey et al., 2007).

Forensic psychologists can conduct research, applying psychological principles to legal and criminal justice issues. While the specific topics may vary, the activities of a forensic research psychologist closely resemble those of any psychologist engaged in research. These activities include proposing projects, applying for and managing grants, collecting and analyzing data, and disseminating findings. Forensic psychologists have a vast array of research topics to explore, including (but not limited to) the following:

- investigating how judges and juries make decisions.
- evaluating the effectiveness of various forensic interventions.
- developing and evaluating assessments for use in FMHA.
- assessing the impact of risk and protective factors on crime and delinquency.
- examining public perception of laws and policies.

After completing research projects in their chosen area of interest, forensic psychologists then disseminate their findings. The primary medium for sharing research findings is peer-reviewed articles, which are published in journals that evaluate the rigor and methodology of a research paper to ensure it reaches a specific standard in the field. However, forensic psychologists also communicate their research to wider audiences through books, trade magazines (e.g., *The Champion*, the magazine of the National Association of Criminal Defense Lawyers), newsletters (e.g., the *American Psychology-Law Society Newsletter*), law review articles, policy briefs, op-eds, and program evaluation reports. Research findings may also be disseminated through presentations, such as those at conferences. These channels allow for a broader reach and impact, further contributing to the development of the field.

CONSULTATION

There are considerable opportunities for forensic psychologists to apply their expertise through consultation. As with every area of practice, the scope of consultation services varies depending on the forensic psychologist's specific area of expertise and background. For example, forensic psychologists specializing in FMHA may be hired by an attorney to review and critique the report of an opposing expert, to help an attorney develop a case strategy, to give opinions on whether the attorney's client followed best practices in a specific context, or to help in jury selection. Those specializing in research can offer consultation on research study methodologies, statistical analyses, and interpretation of results. Further, psychologists may be asked to testify regarding their areas of subject matter expertise in court, such as providing testimony on general factors that can influence eyewitness memory or that can influence a defendant providing a false confession.

KNOW THE LINGO

Forensic psychologists who evaluate an individual and provide opinion testimony regarding that individual's clinical functioning as it relates to a psycholegal question are called *evaluative experts*. In contrast, experts who testify based on their subject matter expertise when it is relevant to a case are called *scientific experts*, alternatively referred to as *teaching experts*. Regardless of whether a psychologist is an evaluative expert or a scientific expert, it is important that they maintain impartiality in their work (ABA, 2016).

Forensic psychologists may consult across different stages of the justice system, addressing areas such as screening and assessment, treatment, and program development or monitoring. With police departments, consultation can be integrated into the police academy to develop mental health assessment and treatment protocols for officers that have experienced job-related trauma or to provide training for officers and emergency medical technicians on interacting with individuals with mental illness or substance use disorders (see Marques & Paulino, 2022). Within the court system, forensic psychologists can assist in the development, analysis, or monitoring of specialized court programs (e.g., community courts, drug courts, mental health courts) (see DeMatteo et al., 2019). In correctional settings, consultation may involve advising on the utilization of appropriate assessment tools and aiding the facility in the development, evaluation, and provision of psychological services (e.g., Stringer, 2019). Forensic psychologists can also provide consultation services to government agencies, offering comprehensive assessments of their systems to identify service gaps or assist with legal and policy matters (e.g., Griffin et al., 2015).

MENTORSHIP, SUPERVISION, AND TEACHING

Forensic psychologists, like many other types of psychologists, may also be involved in mentorship, supervision, and teaching. These roles can assume various forms (formal and informal) and cater to any career stage, including prospective students, graduate students, postdoctoral fellows, early-career professionals, and seasoned experts. By actively engaging in these activities, forensic psychologists contribute to the advancement of the field by fostering career growth and supporting the next generation of psychologists.

As mentors, forensic psychologists play a pivotal role in guiding and shaping the development of others in the field. The more traditional approach to mentorship in forensic psychology involves a faculty advisor and a graduate student. In many Ph.D. programs, students apply to a program to work with and be mentored by a specific faculty member. The mentor's responsibilities include providing guidance throughout the student's training, assisting in research projects, offering course selection advice, and providing professional and personal support (Johnson, 2014). Mentorship can also occur more informally, such as meeting with an early-career professional over coffee or a quick phone call to provide professional advice (APA, 2006).

Supervision is another important component of developing the skillset and careers of others in the field. It may involve formal supervision of clinical hours, particularly before licensure, or it can encompass a broader scope where individuals teach and train others. In clinical treatment and assessment, licensed psychologists can oversee the work of other non–licensed clinicians (e.g., doctoral students in psychology). The supervision entails guiding cases, reviewing clinical documentation, supporting professional development, promoting evidence-based approaches and best practices, and upholding ethical and legal standards (Falender & Shafranske, 2014). Through effective supervision, forensic psychologists ensure the delivery of high-quality services and maintain the integrity of the field. Supervision can also occur in the other areas described in this book, such as supervising research, policy work, or teaching.

Teaching and instruction are also integral aspects of forensic psychology. Many forensic psychologists assume teaching roles, imparting their knowledge and expertise to others. Professors at academic institutions teach general psychology courses or specialized courses in forensic psychology to undergraduate and/or graduate students. The specific courses taught may vary depending on each individual's subarea of expertise (e.g., clinical, research methodology, developmental, neuropsychology). Still, the overall activities generally include developing a course, providing weekly lectures, designing and grading assignments, and cultivating student learning, both within and beyond the confines of the classroom (Forsyth, 2016). Forensic psychologists also teach in diverse settings and to various audiences. This may involve instructing other psychologists with continuing education, teaching behavioral didactics at medical schools, or educating the legal system on the behavioral sciences.

GATEKEEPING

In many fields, including psychology, gatekeeping acts as a filter for quality standards and ethics. Forensic psychologists should only engage in the professional activities for which they are adequately trained and qualified. Gatekeepers in forensic psychology contribute to maintaining the integrity and professionalism of the field. In clinical practice, gatekeepers ensure those who practice are qualified and well-trained. This could entail developing professional and ethical guidelines and ensuring that standards of practice are clearly laid out. Additionally, gatekeepers may serve on boards overseeing the licensure or board certification process, carefully evaluating the qualifications of those who apply. Further, gatekeeping can happen on a microlevel; clinical practitioners may gatekeep within their organization or practice to ensure they uphold ethical standards (Homrich, 2018). From a research perspective, gatekeepers serve as the critical evaluators who determine which grants receive funding, which research protocols are approved (e.g., serving on an Institutional Review Board), which presentations are accepted to research conferences, and which studies get published. Their expertise and discernment ensure that only high-quality and rigorous research contributes to the advancement of forensic psychology.

It is important to acknowledge that gatekeeping is a complex and nuanced topic. Poorly executed gatekeeping practices can inadvertently contribute to disparities within the field, limit opportunities, or perpetuate biases. Therefore, it is crucial for gatekeeping activities to be conducted with careful consideration to enhance the integrity of the field.

POLICY

Forensic psychologists can play a significant role in shaping policy and law by applying their expertise in psychology and the legal system. They contribute to policy through various outlets, including evaluating existing policy, planning new policy initiatives, consulting with policymakers, and assessing public perception of policy-related matters. These activities can occur within a government institution, non-profit organization, through independently conducted policy-relevant studies, or through other policy-relevant scholarship and writing.

FORENSIC FUN FACT

Psychologists have been integral in reshaping punishment approaches for individuals with mental health challenges, as well as for juvenile offenders. For example, the American Psychological Association submitted *amicus curiae* (friend of the court) briefs in *Atkins v. Virginia* (2002), *Roper v. Simmons* (2005), and *Miller v. Alabama* (2012). Respectively, these Supreme Court cases had the effect of abolishing the death penalty for defendants with an Intellectual Disability; abolishing the death penalty for juvenile offenders; and abolishing mandatory life without parole sentences for juvenile offenders.

Forensic psychologists can shape public policy by leveraging their research into advocacy efforts. Their research may inform the development of new policies by providing evidence on factors that influence behavior, public attitudes, and potential consequences of different policy options. For example, researchers may investigate the underlying factors related to criminal behavior, which can inform the development of policies focused on deflection, diversion, and treatment. Additionally, they can evaluate the effectiveness of existing policies and assess their impact on specific communities.

Moreover, forensic psychologists engage in advocacy efforts to promote policy change. One impactful method is through the submission of *amicus curiae* briefs. *Amicus curiae* briefs are legal documents filed by individuals or entities who are not directly involved in a case but who possess valuable insights that can inform the court's decision. The APA occasionally writes and submits amicus briefs to leverage expertise to influence policy, articulating to the court how a specific policy or outcome aligns with research and evidence-based practices. They may include relevant research and data, ethical considerations, and implications for practice. The APA maintains an *amicus curiae* brief program, which has submitted over 200 briefs, several of which have been cited by the Supreme Court and influenced judicial decisions (DeAngelis, 2019). Most notably, psychologists filed a brief in *Brown v. Board of Education* (1954), informing the court of psychological research findings on the harmful effects of racial discrimination. APA briefs have also been influential in cases regarding gender discrimination (*Price Waterhouse v. Hopkins,* 1989), disability rights (*Atkins v. Virginia,* 2002), and false confessions (*Warney v. State of New York,* 2011), among others (DeAngelis, 2019).

CASE LAW REVIEW

In *Brown v. Board of Education* (1954), a landmark case that ended racial segregation in public schools, the Supreme Court drew heavily on contributions from psychological science. The Court noted, "To separate [Black students] from others of similar age and qualifications solely because of their race generates a feeling of inferiority as to their status in the community that may affect their hearts and minds in a way unlikely ever to be undone" (p. 494). Therefore, the Court stated, "Separate educational facilities are inherently unequal" (p. 495). As such, the Court held that racial segregation in schools violated the Fourteenth Amendment's Equal Protection Clause.

CHAPTER TAKEAWAYS

Forensic psychologists engage in various professional activities that align with the broader field of psychology but with a focus on addressing legal issues and questions. Forensic psychologists offer services across the various stages of the justice system, utilizing research, clinical practice, and consultation to inform and influence legal decision making. Forensic psychologists also shape the development of aspiring psychologists in the field with supervision, mentorship, and teaching. You now know what the field of forensic psychology is, as well as the common career activities that forensic psychologists engage in. But in what career settings can you ply the trade of forensic psychology? Turn the page to find out!

REFERENCES

American Bar Association. (2016). *Criminal justice standards on mental health* (4th ed.). https://www.americanbar.org/content/dam/aba/publications/criminal_justice_ standards/mental_health_standards_2016.pdf

American Psychological Association. (2006). *Introduction to mentoring: A guide for mentors and mentees.* https://www.apa.org/education-career/grad/mentoring

American Psychological Association. (2013). Specialty guidelines for forensic psychology. *American Psychologist, 68*(1), 7–19. https://doi.org/10.1037/a0029889

American Psychological Association. (2022). *APA guidelines for child custody evaluations in family law proceedings.* https://www.apa.org/about/policy/child-custody-evaluations.pdf

American Psychology Association. (2018). Professional practice guidelines for occupationally mandated psychological evaluations. *American Psychologist, 73*(2), 186–197. http://dx.doi.org/10.1037/amp0000170

Atkins v. Virginia, 536 U.S. 304 (2002).

Bonta, J., & Andrews, D. A. (2023). *The psychology of criminal conduct* (7th ed.). Routledge. https://doi.org/10.4324/9781003292128

Brown v. Board of Education, 347 U.S. 483 (1954).

Craig, L. A., Dixon, L., & Gannon, T. A. (2013). *What works in offender rehabilitation: An evidence-based approach to assessment and treatment.* Wiley. http://dx.doi.org/10.1002/9781118320655

DeAngelis, T. (2019). Informing the courts with the best research. *Monitor on Psychology, 50*(11), 48. https://www.apa.org/monitor/2019/12/cover-courts

DeMatteo, D., Fairfax-Columbo, J., & Desai, A. (2020). *Becoming a forensic psychologist.* Routledge.

DeMatteo, D., Heilbrun, K., Thornewill, A., & Arnold, A. (2019). *Problem-solving courts and the criminal justice system.* Oxford University Press. https://psycnet.apa.org/doi/10.1093/med-psych/9780190844820.001.0001

Dusky v. United States, 362 U.S. 402 (1960).

Falender, C. A., & Shafranske, E. P. (2014). Clinical supervision and the era of competence. In W. B. Johnson & N. K. Kaslow (Eds.), *The oxford handbook of education and training in professional psychology.* Oxford University Press.

Forsyth, D. R. (2016). *College teaching: Practical insights from the science of teaching and learning.* American Psychological Association. http://dx.doi.org/10.1037/14777-001

Griffin, P. A., LaDuke, C., Abreu, D., Winckworth-Prejsnar, K., Filone, S., Dorrell, S., & Finello, C. (2015). Using the Sequential Intercept Model in cross-systems mapping. In P. A. Griffin, K. Heilbrun, E. P. Mulvey, D. DeMatteo, & C. A. Schubert (Eds.), *The Sequential Intercept Model and criminal justice.* Oxford University Press. https://psycnet.apa.org/doi/10.4324/9781315627823-19

Grossi, L. M., Cabeldue, M., & Brereton, A. (2021). Cognitive behavior therapy for psychosis (CBT-p) as an adjunct to competency restoration. *Journal of Forensic Psychology Research and Practice, 21*(4), 317–337. https://doi.org/10.1080/24732850.2021.1877022

Heilbrun, K., DeMatteo, D., Brooks Holliday, S., & LaDuke, C. (Eds.). (2014). *Forensic mental health assessment: A casebook* (2nd ed.). Oxford University Press. https://psycnet.apa.org/doi/10.1093/med:psych/9780199941551.001.0001

Heilbrun, K., Giallella, C., Wright, H. J., DeMatteo, D., Griffin, P. A., Locklair, B., & Desai, A. (2019). Treatment for restoration of competence to stand trial: Critical analysis and policy recommendations. *Psychology, Public Policy, and Law, 25*(4), 266–283. https://doi.org/10.1037/law0000210

Heilbrun, K., Grisso, T., & Goldstein, A. (2009). *Foundations of forensic mental health assessment.* Oxford University Press.

Homrich, A. M. (2018). Introduction to gatekeeping. In A. M. Homrich & K. L. Henderson (Eds.), *Gatekeeping in the mental health professions.* American Counseling Association.

Huss, M. T. (2014). *Forensic psychology: Research, clinical practice, and applications.* Wiley.

Jackson v. Indiana, 406 U.S. 715 (1972).

Johnson, B. W. (2014). Mentoring in psychology education and training: A mentoring relationship continuum model. In W. B. Johnson & N. K. Kaslow (Eds.), *The Oxford handbook of education and training in professional psychology*. Oxford University Press.

Kane, A. W., & Dvoskin, J. (2011). *Evaluation for personal injury claims*. Oxford University Press.

Kim, B., Benekos, P. J., & Merlo, A. V. (2016). Sex offender recidivism revisited: Review of recent meta-analyses on the effects of sex offender treatment. *Trauma, Violence, & Abuse*, 17(1), 105–117. https://doi.org/10.1177/1524838014566719

Lipsey, M. W., Landenberger, N. A., & Wilson, S. J. (2007). Effects of cognitive-behavioral programs for criminal offenders. *Campbell Systematic Reviews*, 6. https://doi.org/10.4073/csr.2007.6

Marques, P. B., & Paulino, M. (2022). *Police psychology: New trends in forensic psychological science*. Elsevier Science & Technology.

Melton, G. B., Petrila, J., Poythress, N. G., Slobogin, C., Otto, R. K., Mossman, D., & Condie, L. O. (2018). *Psychological evaluation for the courts: A handbook for mental health professionals and lawyers* (4th ed.). The Guilford Press.

Monahan, J., & Skeem, J. L. (2016). Risk assessment in criminal sentencing. *Annual Review of Clinical Psychology*, 12, 489–513. https://doi.org/10.1146/annurev-clinpsy-021815-092945

Munetz, M. R., & Griffin, P. A. (2006). Use of the Sequential Intercept Model as an approach to decriminalization of people with serious mental illness. *Psychiatric Services*, 57(4), 544–549. https://doi.org/10.1176/ps.2006.57.4.544

Price Waterhouse v. Hopkins, 490 U.S. 228 (1989).

Reeves, B. A. (2012). *Hiring and retention of state and local law enforcement officers, 2008- Statistical Tables*. Bureau of Justice Statistics, U.S. Department of Justice.

Stringer, H. (2019). Improving mental health for inmates. *Monitor on Psychology*, 50(3), 46. https://www.apa.org/monitor/2019/03/mental-heath-inmates

Warney v. State of New York, 16 N.Y.3d 428 (2011).

Zapf, P. A., & Roesch, R. (2009). *Evaluation of competence to stand trial*. Oxford University Press.

CHAPTER 3

Okay . . . So What Types of Settings Can Forensic Psychologists Work In?

By the time you are nearing the end of your graduate education and training, you will have amassed a strong, varied skillset that has prepared you for numerous settings. As a result, many work environments will be available for you to pursue based on your expertise, career goals, desired professional activities, and interests, not to mention factors such as work-life balance. So, the question becomes: When you picture yourself commuting into the office (or in a post-COVID world, walking over to your kitchen-turned-office five minutes after your alarm goes off) for a day of work, what image comes to mind?

In this chapter, we introduce the primary settings in which forensic psychologists work, including the types of professional roles associated with each. We hope that this chapter will help you to start crystallizing the image of yourself as a forensic mental health professional. Whether you are preparing for your first forensic job or looking to pivot from the setting in which you have been working, this chapter also provides an idea of the types of professional skills to hone to best position yourself for a job in your ideal setting.

THE FUNDAMENTAL FORENSIC WORKPLACES

Although there are exceptions, forensic mental health professionals' workplaces typically map onto three realms: academic, clinical, and policy-focused. For some of you, the setting you are most interested in will be dictated by the types of professional activities you hope to engage in throughout your career. For others, the setting itself will be the draw, directing your pursuit of

DOI: 10.4324/9781003408857-4

training in the relevant competencies. As you familiarize yourself with these three settings, bear in mind that there may be opportunities for overlap in professional realms or activities.

The Academic Workplace

If you spent your college years inspired by the classrooms and campus or found yourself thinking, "That's the life I want," when you first encountered Professor Gerald Lambeau in *Good Will Hunting*, chances are you may be drawn to academic workplaces. For forensic psychologists, this consists of post-secondary education, such as colleges and universities. Although most academic settings are unlikely to consistently match the intensity of that portrayed in an award-winning film or the wonder of a particularly beautiful fall day on campus, academic settings offer fulfilling and diverse careers in forensic psychology. Exactly how a job in academia looks varies widely across location, type of school, and department (explored in depth in forthcoming chapters). Further, the academic setting most suited for a forensic mental health professional may depend on their degree.

One of the primary distinctions among academic workplaces is that of undergraduate- or graduate-level universities. As with most professional settings, having a doctoral degree (Ph.D. or Psy.D.) will equip you with the qualifications needed for the broadest range of academic settings, including doctoral programs. In contrast, master's-level forensic mental health professionals may be more likely to secure an academic position in an undergraduate or master's program.

Within undergraduate programs, forensic psychologists often will be housed in the Psychology Department. However, given the intersectional nature of forensic psychology, there may be opportunities for positions within other departments, such as Criminal Justice or Criminology. This will depend on the existence of such departments within the universities you are considering and the specifics of your training and expertise. For example, a forensic psychologist with a primarily clinical background (e.g., Psy.D.) may be more suited for a role within the Psychology Department, whereas someone who focused on non-clinical research and criminal justice reform during their graduate training and early career may be more suited for a Criminology Department position. Within graduate universities, forensic psychologists may be hired into master's and/or doctoral (Ph.D. or Psy.D.) programs. However, even if hired into a position housed within a graduate program, roles and responsibilities may overlap with undergraduate settings, such as teaching undergraduate courses or mentoring undergraduate students.

Regardless of department or academic level, forensic psychologists are likely to enter an academic professional setting as a junior faculty member and advance through promotion and tenure across positions: assistant professor, associate professor, and full professor. There also may be opportunities to pursue academic leadership positions, such as Director of Clinical Training, Department Chair, Dean, or Provost. Whereas professors are centered on teaching and mentorship, leadership positions often involve management and oversight, administrative responsibilities, and program planning and implementation.

Professional Activities in the Academic Realm

Forensic psychologists who work in academic settings will typically participate in a range of professional activities: teaching, mentoring or advising trainees and junior colleagues, securing grant funding and conducting research, and publishing. Service roles, such as committee member within the university or peer reviewer for an academic journal, also may be expected in an academic setting. Further, because forensic psychologists receive clinical training and education, those working in graduate-level academic settings may have opportunities for clinical work, such as providing supervision within a clinic staffed by pre-doctoral trainees (e.g., a university-based psychological services center).

FORENSIC FUN FACT

Psychologists have been increasingly likely to assume academic leadership positions in recent years. From 2003 to 2015, there was a 61% increase in psychologists in faculty positions securing leadership roles (American Psychological Association, 2020). These changes have been observed across demographic groups, including women and Black, Indigenous, and People of Color (BIPOC) psychologists (American Psychological Association, 2020).

As highlighted, working in an academic setting provides rich opportunities for a variety of professional activities, particularly if housed within a doctoral program. The exact breakdown and presence of these activities will depend on the setting and the contract you negotiate with your employers. Regarding differences by setting, the graduate program's training model provides insight into the specific roles that may be expected for an academic position. Specifically, doctoral-level psychology programs typically follow one of two training approaches: scientist-practitioner or practitioner-scholar (explored in more detail in Chapter 5). Whereas a scientist-practitioner model equally emphasizes conducting research and delivering mental health treatment, a practitioner-scholar model focuses more on applying research to clinical practice than on conducting research (Stoltenberg et al., 2000). Therefore, forensic psychologists who work in scientist-practitioner graduate programs may be more likely to mentor student research projects and write grants, for example, than those working in practitioner-scholar programs.

FORENSIC FUN FACT

In a survey of academic clinical psychologists, Himelein and Putnam (2001) found that psychologists' responsibilities primarily consisted of teaching undergraduate or graduate courses (37%), followed by conducting and overseeing research (26%) and conducting clinical work (12%), such as providing mental health treatment and supervising trainees (Himelein & Putnam, 2001). The type of academic setting also impacted the emphasis on specific roles. Specifically, the faculty of Ph.D. programs reported dedicating the greatest amount of time to research, whereas the faculty at undergraduate and master's-level programs reported allocating the most time to teaching (Himelein & Putnam, 2001).

A Final Note on Academic Settings

Just as college campuses differ significantly in their look and feel, the specific professional activities of a forensic psychologist working in an academic setting will differ. Because of the diversity of these activities, academic settings are unlikely to follow a traditional "9-to-5" work schedule. Working on nights and weekends may be common. Additionally, although campuses may clear out over summer and winter breaks—and with it, your teaching responsibilities—year-round expectations for research, mentorship, and scholarship remain.

The Clinical Workplace

Others of you may envision a career in which no two days are the same, each spent working with clients who present with different mental health needs, assisting the legal system by assessing legally involved individuals who may be experiencing mental health symptoms, or supervising the next generation of forensic mental health professionals. You may picture yourself stepping out to a clinic waiting room to welcome a patient into your office or consulting closely with interdisciplinary teams on your caseload. If this describes you, welcome to the clinical realm of forensic practice.

Like other mental health jobs, forensic clinical work often occurs in hospital-based inpatient units or outpatient clinics, community-based mental health clinics, or private practice. However, due to the unique overlap with the legal system, forensic psychologists also may work in correctional settings, law enforcement settings, or in conjunction with courts. Within each of these clinical settings, a great deal of variety exists. As a saying among clinicians who work in Veterans Affairs Medical Centers (VAMC) goes, "When you've seen one VA, you've seen one VA." This adage likely applies to the entire spectrum of clinical workplaces.

Hospital-based work settings for forensic psychologists include academic or university-affiliated medical centers, psychiatric hospitals, and VAMCs. Some psychiatric hospitals—such as state hospitals, forensic hospitals, or public hospitals with specialized forensic units (e.g., New York City's Bellevue Hospital Center)—have a specific forensic focus and work closely with the local criminal legal system.

Outside of hospitals, forensic psychologists may work in community mental health settings that focus on mental health needs associated with legal involvement. For example, these clinics may specialize in the treatment of substance use disorder or intimate partner violence. Finally, clinical doctoral programs often have some form of a psychology clinic where doctoral students receive practicum training, which offers an additional environment in which forensic psychologists may work. Of note, university-based clinical settings likely overlap with academic appointments. One such example is the Drexel Reentry Project (DRP) housed within Drexel University's Psychological Services Center. The DRP was developed in partnership with the Supervision to Aid Reentry (STAR) Program, a federal reentry court in Philadelphia, Pennsylvania. This service provides skills-based cognitive behavioral therapy (CBT) to individuals who were previously incarcerated and are participating in the STAR Program (Heilbrun et al., 2017). Mental health treatment is provided by pre-doctoral clinical psychology students (practicum students), who are supervised by a licensed forensic psychologist with an academic appointment in Drexel University's Department of Psychological and Brain Sciences. Over the years, as needs within the community have evolved, the Drexel Reentry Project has continued to grow to include mental health interventions for exonerees (Heilbrun et al., 2022).

Uniquely, forensic psychologists may work in clinical settings within the criminal legal system, such as correctional facilities, courts, or law enforcement agencies. In these settings, forensic psychologists provide treatment to and conduct assessments of individuals who are legally involved and experiencing mental health challenges. Forensic psychologists also may secure court-based or court-affiliated appointments. For example, they may be housed within a problem-solving court to receive referrals and provide rehabilitative mental health services to court participants. They may also work within police departments, the Federal Bureau of Investigation

(FBI), or the Central Intelligence Agency (CIA). Still, other examples of government-affiliated clinical settings exist, such as state Departments of Health and Human Services.

Finally, forensic psychologists who pursue a clinical career may, in effect, create their own workplace via a solo or group private practice. Some private practitioners may partner with problem-solving courts for mandated treatment and meet with their clients in an outpatient office setting. Those who primarily conduct forensic mental health assessments may enjoy more of a dynamic, traveling office, where evaluations are conducted in their office, a lawyer's office, a court, or a correctional facility depending on the case and the evaluee's disposition (e.g., pre-trial, incarcerated, on probation) at the time of the evaluation.

FORENSIC FUN FACT

Problem-solving courts link justice-involved individuals to mental health and psychosocial services to address unmet needs (e.g., substance use disorder, unemployment) that may contribute to criminal behavior and recidivism. Participant progress is monitored through regular attendance at court sessions with a judge, communication with parole and probation officers, and urine drug testing. Problem-solving courts may serve as an alternative to incarceration, as in the case of drug court or veterans courts, or can offer reductions to length of parole, as in the case of reentry courts (Miller et al., 2020).

Professional Activities in the Clinical Realm

Regardless of the exact setting, forensic psychologists who work in clinical environments typically provide individual or group-based mental health treatment, conduct forensic mental health assessments, write assessment reports, and in some cases, supervise trainees or junior colleagues. These clinical services may be provided to individuals who are charged, convicted, or incarcerated within the legal system or others who intersect with the legal system, such as victims or witnesses of crimes and law enforcement agents. At times, there may be additional opportunities for diversification of roles and responsibilities, namely, developing clinical programming.

However, just as workplaces within the clinical realm are diverse, the specific nature of these activities differs, and some environments are more likely to present certain professional opportunities. For example, forensic psychologists who work in forensic psychiatric hospitals commonly assess and treat competency to stand trial. Within law enforcement agencies, forensic psychologists' responsibilities can include expert testimony and research or analysis of criminal behavior of suspects, as well as pre-employment and fitness for duty evaluations of law enforcement agents. Still other forensic psychologists may provide training and consultation to lawyers, as well as law enforcement officers and agents. In government settings, forensic clinicians may be responsible for accommodating court orders for assessment or treatment. Within the Colorado Department of Human Services' Forensic Services Department, for example, this includes providing case management for individuals who are found not guilty by reason of insanity (NGRI) and are returning to the community, conducting evaluations of competency to stand trial, and providing competency restoration services (Office of Civil and Forensic Mental Health, n.d.). Rather than working solely out of a correctional facility or correctional mental health institution, these forensic psychologists may be based in the community but serve a similar function within the field of forensic psychology.

FORENSIC FUN FACT

Forensic mental health assessments (FMHA) are comprehensive psychological evaluations that assist legal decision making. FMHA consist of clinical and scientific data drawn from psychological testing, behavioral assessment, self-report, observation, and medical and legal records. Examples of legal questions that can be informed by FMHA include competency to stand trial, mental state at the time of the offense, sentencing, civil commitment, and personal injury, among others (Heilbrun et al., 2009).

A Final Note on Clinical Settings

Even though no two clinical workdays are the same because of differing clients and clinical presentations, this type of workplace may be more suited for those of you who enjoy having your day charted out for you with set professional activities. Whereas academic settings may follow more of a "choose-your-own-adventure" approach to work schedules and responsibilities, clinical work is inherently structured because of a need to schedule clients and appointments. In some hospital or correctional clinical settings in particular, forensic psychologists may encounter shift work that rotates across time of day and days of the week. Particularly in inpatient settings where patient coverage is a constant need, working the occasional weekend or holiday may be expected.

The Policy-Focused Workplace

Although it might not be the first thing that comes to mind when picturing the workplace of a forensic psychologist, some of you may be most excited by the "standard" office. Here, days are primarily spent at a desk, with colleagues down the hall ready to brainstorm ideas, commiserate over work, or ideally, do both while taking a coffee break. Despite the portrayals of this type of workplace in films like *Office Space*, many people thrive in this environment. (For the record, we do not condone the destruction of office property.) If this describes you—even without the promise of taking out your frustration on unsuspecting printers—you may value a policy-focused role.

Policy-focused forensic work can occur in a number of settings. Individuals who work for government agencies can operate at the county, state, or federal level, such as county or state Departments of Behavioral Health or the United States Department of Veterans Affairs. Further, forensic-focused policy work can occur in think tanks, non-profit organizations, and nongovernmental organizations (NGOs) with a criminal justice focus. One example is the RAND Corporation (www.rand.org), a non-profit, research-focused organization that aims to inform solutions to public policy issues, including justice and the criminal legal system.

Professional Activities in the Policy Realm

Policy-focused organizations concentrate on shaping and evaluating laws and practices concerning forensic mental health. Professional activities that are particularly suited for this type of forensic work include informing organizations and governments on policies impacting individuals with mental health issues and justice involvement. This may take the form of proposing and analyzing legislation and regulations, engaging in advocacy efforts and testifying to committees, developing and evaluating programs and continuous quality improvement, and researching or evaluating the effectiveness of new policies to inform an evidence-based approach. In recent years, greater focus has turned to forensic policy that establishes collaborations between law enforcement and mental health providers, such as co-responder teams, police-assisted diversion from arrest (also called deflection), and crisis intervention team training. Other policy-focused initiatives include efforts to improve rehabilitative services for individuals who are reentering the community following incarceration, promote harm reduction initiatives for substance abuse, facilitate pardons of previous convictions, and expunge records.

KNOW THE LINGO

Police-assisted diversion, or *deflection*, focuses on diversion from *arrest*. In lieu of arresting an individual, law enforcement officers refer individuals to treatment and social support resources in the community. This allows individuals to be connected to stabilizing services while preventing them from formally entering the criminal justice system (Charlier, 2015).

A NOTE ON ROLE DIVERSIFICATION

Although we have provided a general framework for distinguishing among these three settings, it is valuable to remember that one of the benefits of comprehensive, doctoral-level training in forensic psychology is the broad range of skills with which you graduate. In other words, for those of you who still envision yourselves walking into a hospital for work every day but now realize that you want to continue contributing to the scientific literature after you have earned your degree, worry not!

As may be clear by this point, overlap in activities exists across forensic work settings. A forensic psychologist who works in an academic setting may be able to contribute equally to the clinical and research realms, particularly within scientist-practitioner doctoral programs. Although it may be less common due to the nature of healthcare and an ever-growing demand for mental health services, it is possible to negotiate protected time for research and publishing in a clinical work setting. This may be particularly true in university-affiliated hospitals or mental health centers given their focus on training and education. Further, in some settings, such as VA Medical Centers, a forensic psychologist may secure a position providing mental health treatment to legally involved veterans, conducting research, influencing policy, or engaging in some combination of these three. It is worth thinking about the type of setting that affords you the *most* consistency with the type of professional activities you hope to engage in and then to proceed accordingly. Further insight into how to decide among work settings will be covered later in this book.

VENTURING BEYOND THE TRADITIONAL OFFICE

The Traveling Office

Just in case we have not provided you with enough food for thought, there is an additional workplace: the traveling office. Forensic psychologists in private practice may spend their workdays in a traditional office setting or in a correctional facility, a municipal building, or if called to testify for a case, a courtroom. Some forensic psychologists have experienced all of these in just one month's time. Further, private practitioners who offer training, conduct program evaluations, or provide consultation services may travel to law enforcement agencies or other organizations during their work week.

Given their advanced level of training, forensic psychologists may be called as expert witnesses or fact witnesses, which can involve creating a make-shift office while waiting to testify in court. As expert witnesses, forensic psychologists are asked to attest to a legal question or issue based on clinical or research background and training (Sageman, 2003). Academic forensic psychologists may be secured as expert witnesses based on their advanced knowledge of a specific research base, such as the impact of alcohol use on cognitive ability. Additionally, clinical forensic psychologists can be asked to serve as an expert witness after completing a forensic mental health assessment; in these cases, they would be asked to provide context relevant to a legal question (e.g., adjudicative competence, mental state at the time of the offense). As a fact witness, forensic mental health professionals are asked to attest to aspects relevant to an ongoing case that they have observed directly, such as a defendant's behavior during a group therapy session that occurred while awaiting trial in a correctional setting. Whereas expert witnesses can provide *opinions* on a legal matter, fact witnesses can speak only to what they have directly observed or witnessed with regards to that specific case (Committee on the Judiciary, 2025).

Work Settings in a Post-COVID World

Okay, it turns out there is one more forensic work setting to mention. (Wondering if this will ever end? How very "2020" of you.) Although these broader work settings still hold, the COVID-19 pandemic has popularized the remote or hybrid workplace. For those of you reading this chapter from said kitchen-turned-office (or in line at the grocery store while clocked in to work [we're not here to judge]), this one's for you.

Many industries have shifted to hybrid or remote workplaces since March 2020. Depending on the organization, these options may be available for research and policy-based forensic work. Although it will largely depend on the college or university, academic roles may offer hybrid opportunities but might require at least some presence on campus as long as students are attending in person. However, although some work environments for forensic psychologists lend themselves well to opportunities for part- and full-time remote work, others may require in-person work. This may be true of clinical work, particularly in inpatient settings, and work within law enforcement agencies, courts, or correctional facilities.

In keeping with the changing landscape of technology and healthcare, the American Psychological Association (APA) has developed *Professional Practice Guidelines for the Practice of Telepsychology* (APA, 2013). Although we are learning and expanding in this realm, particularly with the mandatory temporary migration to remote provision of care during the COVID-19 pandemic, forensic mental health assessments may continue to require some degree of in-person work, as the validity of certain measures is contingent on in-person administration. Within the broader field of psychology, forensic mental health is still developing its understanding of the feasibility of telepsychology. However, there is already support for the electronic or online administration of some commonly used measures in forensic mental health assessment, such as the Minnesota Multiphasic Personality Inventory (MMPI) series and the Personality Assessment Inventory (PAI) (Kois et al., 2021), and the American Psychology-Law Society (AP-LS) maintains updated telepsychology resources for forensic practitioners (https://ap-ls.org/resources/telepsychology/telepsychology.html). Further research on important considerations related to FMHA, such as the impact of using videoconferencing for clinical interviewing on evaluee perceptions of privacy, is necessary to establish that telepsychology is commensurate to in-person interactions in forensic contexts (Kois et al., 2021).

Nonetheless, the COVID-19 pandemic introduced increased flexibility in clinical work settings as well, including the expansion of laws regulating clinical practice. For example, the Psychology Interjurisdictional Compact (PSYPACT; www.psypact.gov/) is an interstate agreement that allows psychologists from participating states to practice across state lines without securing licensure in said state. This has permitted psychologists to work from home offices in one state while meeting with clients who reside in another state. Some of these aspects governing clinical work will remain, but other changes may be temporary. Therefore, it is always important to familiarize yourself with the laws and guidelines governing forensic work in the states in which you intend to work.

CHAPTER TAKEAWAYS

Now that you have learned about different professional settings for forensic mental health professionals, return to the image of yourself preparing for a day of work. The image in your mind may be clearer than ever, or you may feel even more overwhelmed by the sheer number of exciting possibilities that will be available to you upon completion of your forensic training and education. The good news is that your career can—and likely will—take many forms over your lifetime, and if you work to keep your diverse skillset sharp regardless of your work environment, you will be able to seek different opportunities throughout your career. Over the coming chapters, we will delve deeper into the various career paths and activities, as well as related decisional factors, which will provide further clarity and direction. For the time being, settle into your seat, look out of your current (or imagined) office window, and entertain the many possible roads ahead!

REFERENCES

American Psychological Association. (2013). Professional practice guidelines for the practice of telepsychology. *American Psychologist, 68*(9), 791–800. https://doi.org/10.1037/a0035001

American Psychological Association. (2020). *Factsheet: Increases in psychologists in academic leadership.* https://www.apa.org/workforce/publications/leadership.pdf

Charlier, J. (2015). Want to reduce drugs in your community? You might want to deflect instead of arrest. *Police Chief Magazine, 82*(9), 30–31. https://www.policechiefmagazine.org/magazine-issues/september-2015/

Committee on the Judiciary. (2025). *Federal rules of evidence.* U.S. Government Publishing Office. https://www.uscourts.gov/sites/default/files/2025-02/federal-rules-of-evidence-dec-1-2024_0.pdf

Heilbrun, K., Grisso, T., & Goldstein, A. M. (2009). *Foundations of forensic mental health assessment.* Oxford University Press.

Heilbrun, K., Pietruszka, V., Thornewill, A., Phillips, S., & Schiedel, R. (2017). Diversion at re-entry using criminogenic CBT: Review and prototypical program development. *Behavioral Sciences & the Law,* 1–11. https://doi.org/10.1002/bsl.2311

Heilbrun, K., Schwartz, J., Wiltsie, K., Lankford, C., Fishel, S., Swenson, A., & Charles, D. (2022). Interventions with individuals exonerated from criminal convictions: Toward development of evidence-based practices in a psychology training clinic. *Practice Innovations.* https://psycnet.apa.org/doi/10.1037/pri0000175

Himelein, M. J., & Putnam, E. A. (2001). Work activities of academic clinical psychologists: Do they practice what they teach? *Professional Psychology: Research and Practice, 32*(5), 537–542. https://psycnet.apa.org/doi/10.1037/0735-7028.32.5.537

Kois, L. E., Cox, J., & Peck, A. T. (2021). Forensic e-mental health: Review, research priorities, and policy directions. *Psychology, Public Policy, and Law, 27*(1), 1–16. https://psycnet.apa.org/doi/10.1037/law0000293

Miller, M. K., Block, L. M., & DeVault, A. (2020). Problem-solving courts in the United States and around the world: History, evaluation, and recommendations. In M. K. Miller & B. H. Bornstein (Eds.), *Advances in psychology and law, Vol. 5* (pp. 301–371). Springer. http://dx.doi.org/10.1007/978-3-030-54678-6_9

Office of Civil and Forensic Mental Health. (n.d.). *Forensic services.* Colorado Department of Human Services. https://cdhs.colorado.gov/behavioral-health/forensic-services

Sageman, M. (2003). Three types of skills for effective forensic psychological assessments. *Assessment, 10*(4), 321–328. https://psycnet.apa.org/doi/10.1177/1073191103259533

Stoltenberg, C. D., Pace, T. M., Kashubeck-West, S., Biever, J. L., Patterson, T., & Welch, I. D. (2000). Training models in counseling psychology: Scientist-practitioner versus practitioner-scholar. *The Counseling Psychologist, 28*(5), 622–640. https://psycnet.apa.org/doi/10.1177/0011000000285002

Part II

Not Just an Ivory Tower

An Exploration of Academic Opportunities in Forensic Psychology

CHAPTER 4

The Perpetual Quest for Knowledge and the Pull to Disseminate

An Overview of Research-Focused Academia

By this point in the book, we hope it is clear that forensic psychologists can do a variety of things in a variety of settings. As we discussed in Chapter 2, given their wide-ranging skills, forensic psychologists can, among other things, conduct forensic mental health assessments and provide forensically relevant treatment (if clinically trained), serve as an expert witness, teach at a college/university, conduct research, disseminate research results (e.g., publications, presentations), mentor and supervise students, and engage in policy-relevant work. In addition to engaging in varied activities, forensic psychologists can ply their trade in several different settings. As we discussed in Chapter 3, forensic psychologists are typically found in academic, clinical, and policy settings, although it is not uncommon for forensic psychologists to work in other settings (e.g., law enforcement).

We provided the foundation for our discussion of career paths in forensic psychology in Chapters 1 through 3, so now we will provide more in-depth information about the various roles and activities of forensic psychologists and the settings in which forensic psychologists often work. Part II of this book (Chapters 4 and 5) will explore academic opportunities in forensic psychology. Specifically, this chapter will discuss research-focused academia, while Chapter 5 will focus on practice-oriented and teaching-oriented academia. As will be discussed, working in academia provides many benefits and opportunities for forensic psychologists. Although it is often quipped that the three best reasons for being in an academic position are June, July, and August, we will discuss some other (less tongue-in-cheek) reasons for pursuing a career in academia.

DOI: 10.4324/9781003408857-6

OVERVIEW OF ACADEMIA

If you are heading to college or are currently in college, or if you have already completed your college education, you probably have some idea of what college professors do. Although professors do many different things, their main activities are (1) teaching, (2) conducting research and producing scholarship, and (3) engaging in service activities to the academic department, college/university, and field. In fact, when professors are being evaluated for tenure and promotion, these are the three performance areas on which those decisions are based.

But the degree to which professors focus on teaching, research, and service activities depends on several factors, including their career status (e.g., assistant professor, associate professor, professor), specific field/subfield of interest, and the type of school at which they work. For example, some schools prioritize teaching and do not have a sufficiently well-developed infrastructure for administering large grants to support research. However, many schools place the most emphasis on the professor's research and scholarly accomplishments when determining if the professor should be granted tenure and/or promoted. Research is highly valued in academic settings because it can generate revenue for the school, enhance the school's reputation, attract prospective students to the school, and contribute to the advancement of the field.

Before getting too deep into our discussion of research academia, it is important to highlight the distinction between colleges and universities (see Ross & Durrani, 2023; Rudolph, 1991). Although most people use those two terms interchangeably, there are some important differences between colleges and universities (Cuellar, 2024). For example, colleges are typically smaller in size (both in terms of student enrollment and class size) than universities. Further, while colleges focus primarily on undergraduate programs (e.g., associate's degree, bachelor's degree), universities offer undergraduate programs and graduate programs (e.g., master's degree, Ph.D.). Another distinction is that colleges can either be standalone institutions (e.g., Haverford College, Williams College) or part of a university. Regarding the latter point, large universities, for example, are typically composed of several colleges (e.g., College of Arts and Sciences, College of Engineering, College of Medicine). Most notably, particularly for the purposes of this chapter, universities tend to place more emphasis on research because many graduate degrees are research-based, which provides more opportunities for students to get research experience.

This chapter will focus on conducting research in academic settings, but for the sake of completeness, we will briefly discuss the two other primary activities in which professors engage—i.e., teaching and service. As institutions of higher learning, the primary mission of colleges and universities involves education/teaching. Forensic psychologists with a Ph.D. are well-positioned to teach students at all levels of higher education, including undergraduate and graduate. (As previously noted, Chapter 5 will discuss teaching-oriented academia.) Faculty members at colleges and universities also engage in a range of service activities. Service is a broad term that is typically defined as service to the academic department (e.g., Department of Psychology), school, field, and sometimes the community. Service to the department may consist of sitting on committees (e.g., curriculum committee, diversity committee, thesis/dissertation committees), student advising, and serving in leadership positions (e.g., Director of Clinical Training, Department Chair). Service to the college or university also includes committee work, although the committees tend to have a large scope (e.g., university tenure and promotion committee, university finance committee). Service to the field encompasses a dizzying array of activities, including membership/leadership in professional organizations, serving as a peer reviewer for manuscripts submitted to peer-reviewed journals, reviewing grant proposals, serving as an external reviewer for tenure and promotion, sitting on committees outside of your academic institution (e.g., professional organizations, steering committee), and conducting site visits (e.g., accreditation of academic programs).

RESEARCH IN ACADEMIA

As briefly discussed in Chapter 2, forensic psychologists are well-equipped to conduct research. The education and training a forensic psychologist receives in their Ph.D. program are heavily focused on research—designing research studies, conducting research, and disseminating research results. As such, forensic psychologists in academic settings often conduct research on a variety of forensically relevant topic areas (see DeMatteo et al., 2020, for a discussion of some research foci). Given the different specialty areas within the field of psychology, including clinical, cognitive, developmental, and social, there are numerous topic areas (with forensic relevance) that can be researched by forensic psychologists in academic settings (see Chapter 1 for a discussion of some of these topic areas).

EXAMPLES OF FORENSIC RESEARCH

- Development and validation of violence risk assessment tools
- Evaluating the effectiveness of interventions to reduce recidivism
- Jury and judicial decision making
- Reliability of eyewitness identification
- Reliability of courtroom testimony by children

The importance of research cannot be overstated. Put simply, scientific research facilitates the acquisition of new knowledge, which is one important way of advancing the field of forensic psychology. In brief, research can be used to describe, explain, and predict, and these goals contribute meaningfully to the field (see Marczyk et al., 2005). More specifically, research has the potential to influence practice and policy. For example, conducting research on the predictive validity of risk assessment measures can change how risk is assessed in various settings (e.g., outpatient, inpatient, correctional) and influence the decisions courts make when assessing someone's risk for future problematic behavior (e.g., antisocial, sexual violence, general violence). Research on the effectiveness of competence restoration therapy can influence the way in which forensic psychiatric hospitals attempt to remediate deficits for someone who has been declared incompetent to stand trial. Research on jury and judicial decision making can, among other things, illustrate the role of implicit bias. There are numerous examples of research studies across a range of topic areas, and this type of research can contribute meaningfully to the improvement of the legal and correctional systems (among other systems) (see Huss, 2013; Skeem et al., 2009, for further discussions of the role and importance of research in forensic psychology).

R1 vs. R2 Institutions

Earlier in the chapter, we noted that different colleges/universities place different degrees of emphasis on research. Some smaller colleges may prioritize teaching and place less emphasis on conducting research, while larger universities may expect all faculty to engage in ongoing research. Reviewing the school's website will often provide useful indications of the degree to which the school focuses on research. There is also a more objective way to assess a school's level of research activity. For more than five decades, the Carnegie Classification of Institutions of Higher Education has provided a framework for categorizing colleges and universities. The Basic Classification classifies schools as R1 institutions (very high research activity) and R2 institutions (high research activity). The way schools are determined to be R1 or R2 (or no classification) is quite involved and beyond the scope of this chapter, but the Carnegie classification framework is set to be updated and simplified in 2025. Whereas classification in prior years looked at several data points, only two factors will be considered in distinguishing R1 from R2 institutions. Specifically, R1 status will be conferred upon schools that have $50 million in research expenditures and grant at least 70 research doctorates. Both R1 and R2 institutions have made considerable research contributions to the field of forensic psychology, as you can see from the Career Profiles for this chapter.

CARNEGIE CLASSIFICATION

R1 Schools (Examples)

- Arizona State University
- Drexel University
- George Mason University
- University of Alabama
- University of Nebraska-Lincoln

R2 Schools (Examples)

- Creighton University
- Florida Institute of Technology
- Fordham University
- Montclair State University
- Sam Houston State University

Types of Research

At this point, you may be wondering: What exactly is research? Are there different types of research? Is research always conducted in a laboratory? Those are important questions (and there are several other important questions we will also address). It is not surprising that questions often arise about the nature of research because research has become much more accessible in recent years. If you skim your favorite online news source, it is likely that at least one headline will mention the results of research. For example: Which diet is best? Which medication works the quickest?

Even though research is much more prevalent and accessible these days, there are many misconceptions about what exactly research is, how research is conducted, and what research can tell us. Importantly, research can take on a variety of forms, ranging from simple questionnaires or telemarketer surveys to scientists working with test tubes in laboratories to highly controlled studies in the real world (Marczyk et al., 2005). Some research studies are relatively unsophisticated and consist entirely of observing a group of people, while other research requires a complex design in which participants are assigned to groups, administered different interventions, and followed over time.

Although there are various ways to categorize research, the basic division is between correlational research and experimental research. Correlational research, as the name implies, is focused on the relationship between two (or more) things. For example, correlational research can be used to see if there is a relationship between height and weight or between age and political ideology. There are numerous variables that can be assessed in correlational research, and demonstrating a relationship between variables can have considerable value. However, correlational research only tells you whether two variables are related, and it does not provide any information on whether one variable caused the other. So experimental research is used when the researcher wants to draw a cause-and-effect conclusion. Through more rigorous research designs involving the random assignment of participants into groups, experimental research can determine whether one variable (e.g., medication) caused another variable (e.g., reduction in depressive symptoms).

This discussion of research designs is necessarily oversimplified. For example, some resources categorize research into experimental, quasi-experimental, and non-experimental, with correlational research falling into the category of non-experimental research and quasi-experimental research involving the use of existing groups (as opposed to experimental research, which involves random assignment into groups). There are numerous resources for those interested in learning more about research design and methodology (e.g., Creswell & Creswell, 2022; Kazdin, 2021; Marczyk et al., 2005).

It should not be surprising that research in forensic psychology, with its variety of subfields and its vast array of topic areas, can take on many forms (see Rosenfeld & Penrod, 2011). For example, a researcher might conduct a correlational study to see if there is a relationship between age and antisocial behavior. The researcher might find, for example, that younger people are more likely to engage in antisocial behavior and that older age is associated with a reduction in such behavior. However, as previously noted, correlational research only shows if there is a relationship between things, with no information on whether one variable caused the other variable. A more informative research study might involve following a group of people over time, which is referred to as longitudinal research, to see if their risk for recidivism changes as they get older. Yet another option is an experimental design, which is useful if the researcher wants to draw a cause-and-effect conclusion. For example, if a researcher is interested in examining the effects of an intervention on risk level, the researcher could use a two-group experimental design in which a group of justice-involved individuals is randomly divided into two groups, with one group receiving the intervention of interest (experimental group) and the other group receiving a different intervention (comparison group).

Correlational and experimental research are the traditional forms of research because they are based on the scientific method—i.e., research questions generate hypotheses that are tested by collecting and analyzing data. But there are several other forms of research that can be (and often are) used by forensic psychologists. For example, rather than conducting a study to examine a topic of interest, researchers can analyze the results of an entire body of research on a particular topic. This is known as a meta-analysis, which is a research/statistical technique for combining data from multiple studies that address a similar research question. There have been many meta-analyses in forensic psychology, including ones on violence risk assessment (e.g., Ogonah et al., 2023; Singh et al., 2011), the effect of the label "psychopathy" on sentencing (Berryessa & Wohlstetter, 2019), the role of youth diversion programs in reducing recidivism (Wilson & Hoge, 2013), and the effectiveness of drug treatment courts (Mitchell et al., 2012).

Some forensic psychology researchers conduct case law reviews to examine court decisions in a particular area. For example, several researchers have examined how courts use (or misuse) the results of certain psychological tests in their decision making, including the Personality Assessment Inventory (Meaux et al., 2022) and the Psychopathy Checklist-Revised (DeMatteo et al., 2014). Other researchers have examined how legislatures have responded to influential court decisions (e.g., Flack et al., 2022). These non-traditional research designs are particularly well-suited to addressing forensic questions.

For several reasons, it can be challenging to conduct some types of forensic research, particularly when working with justice-involved individuals. Some of the populations with whom we work are difficult to access, such as jail/prison inmates and adolescents in juvenile detention centers. The Code of Federal Regulations, which is governing law throughout the United States, requires that "vulnerable populations" be given special consideration in research contexts due to concerns about exploitation and coercion (Protection of Human Subjects, 2009). The category of vulnerable populations includes (among others) children, pregnant women, individuals with impaired decision making capacity, and prisoners. Of note, the category "prisoners" is defined broadly to include anyone who is involuntarily confined or detained, including those who are court-mandated to correctional, psychiatric, residential, or treatment settings (see Pirelli et al., 2017; Protection of Human Subjects, 2009). Individuals with intrinsic or extrinsic vulnerability factors tend to be overrepresented in forensic settings, so forensic researchers need to be aware of the laws that govern their research and understand how to disclose and reduce the risk to these populations. These considerations also highlight the importance (and requirement) of obtaining approval to conduct research from an ethics review board (often called an institutional review board (IRB)) (see DeMatteo et al., in press, for a discussion of ethical and legal considerations in forensic research).

Research Funding

Just as there are many types of research designs and many research questions, there is also variety in terms of whether and how research is funded. Some research is not associated with costs per se. For example, although it takes time and effort to conduct a case law review or statutory review, there is no monetary cost to that type of research. Some research, such as administering an online survey, is relatively inexpensive. In that type of research, there may be minimal costs associated with accessing a particular mailing list and providing a small amount of compensation for participants to complete the survey. Other research, however, may involve purchasing costly testing equipment, hiring research personnel, providing generous (but not coercive) compensation to research participants, and buying specialized statistical software. That type of research can cost millions of dollars.

So where does research money come from? Sometimes researchers at academic institutions pay for the cost of research using money they received as part of a start-up package when they were hired. Typically, when someone is hired as a professor, they receive some money (and other things, like lab space and materials) to help them get started with their research. If a researcher no longer has start-up money (or did not receive any), they may use some professional development money to fund their research. Some schools provide a small amount of money to professors each year that can be used for "professional development," which includes research, materials, paying students, etc.

Start-up money and professional development money may be adequate for small research projects, but bigger studies with bigger budgets require bigger sources of funding. This is where grants are useful. Grants are provided by a variety of entities, both federal and state and public and private. There are several federal entities that provide grants. For example, the National Institutes of Health (NIH), which is part of the U.S. Department of Health and Human Services, provides grants to researchers through its 27 institutes and centers (National Institutes of Health, n.d.). Forensic researchers interested in studying something related to drug abuse may seek funding from the National Institute on Drug Abuse (NIDA), while researchers interested in studying mental health may seek funding from the National Institute of Mental Health (NIMH), both of which are institutes under the NIH umbrella. The Substance Abuse and Mental Health Services Administration (SAMHSA, n.d.), which is also an agency within the U.S. Department of Health and Human Services, provides grants for researchers interested in studying behavioral health (e.g., substance use, mental health), among other things. Forensic researchers might also seek funding from the National Science Foundation (NSF, n.d.) (particularly the Law and Science Program), which is an independent federal agency that supports science and engineering. One last example is the National Institute of Justice (NIJ, n.d.), which is the research, development, and evaluation agency of the U.S. Department of Justice. There are also state grants that are useful for forensic researchers, and these are often offered by a commission (e.g., Pennsylvania Commission on Crime and Delinquency) or a state agency (e.g., Pennsylvania Department of Health).

FORENSIC FUN FACT

The U.S. Department of Justice houses the Office of Justice Programs (OJP, n.d.). Each component of the Office of Justice Programs contains grant funding opportunities relevant to forensic psychologists. They include the following:

- Bureau of Justice Assistance
- Bureau of Justice Statistics
- National Institute of Justice
- Office of Juvenile Justice and Delinquency Prevention
- Office for Victims of Crime
- Office of Sex Offender Sentencing, Monitoring, Apprehending, Registering, and Tracking

In addition to federal and state grants, there are a variety of private foundations and professional organizations that provide research money. For example, in terms of private entities, forensic researchers can consider the Annie E. Casey Foundation, Laura and John Arnold Foundation, Pew Charitable Trusts, Spencer Foundation, and William T. Grant Foundation, among many others. Professional organizations, including the American Academy of Forensic Psychology (AAFP) and the American Psychology-Law Society (AP-LS; Division 41 of APA), also provide funding for forensically relevant research.

We only provided a brief overview of grants because grant funding is a complicated topic for several reasons. First, there are different grant mechanisms for different types of research. If your study is a preliminary study, you would be best suited to look for a grant mechanism that is specifically intended to fund pilot research (e.g., NIH R21). A larger study with a bigger budget would need a different grant mechanism, such as the NIH R01. Second, grant budgets can be challenging to create (and challenging to understand!). Many grant mechanisms distinguish between direct costs and indirect costs. Direct costs are for activities or services related to a specific project. Direct costs might include salaries for research staff, training sessions, research materials and equipment, compensation for research participants, and study-specific travel costs. By contrast, indirect costs are for activities or services that benefit more than one project. Stated differently, indirect costs are those costs that are incurred for common or joint objectives and they cannot be specifically identified with a particular project. Sometimes indirect costs are called overhead costs or facilities and administrative costs (F&A). Whereas direct costs are used to conduct a study, indirect costs are given to the organization in which the research is being conducted. This is one reason universities encourage grant-funded research. To further complicate things, some grant funders do not provide indirect costs, and different sponsors have different indirect cost rates.

NIH GRANT MECHANISMS (EXAMPLES)

- R01: Research Project Grant
- R03: Small Grant
- R21: Exploratory

Developmental Grant

- R34: Clinical Trial Planning
- R41/42: Small Business Technology Transfer
- R56: High-Priority, Short-Term Project
- K99: Pathway to Independence Award

SCHOLARSHIP: DISSEMINATING RESEARCH RESULTS

Once research is completed, an important next step is disseminating the results of the research, which is important for two reasons. First, have you ever heard the phrase "publish or perish"? Although it is perhaps a bit dramatic, this phrase emphasizes the importance of publishing in the career of an academic. As we previously noted, one of the performance areas in which professors are evaluated when it comes to tenure and promotion decisions is research and scholarship. Without a sufficient record of research and scholarship—and the definition of "sufficient" varies by school, field, and several other factors—a professor may not be awarded tenure and promoted through the academic ranks. So, disseminating research results has value for a faculty member's career trajectory.

Second, research would have limited value if no one other than the researchers knew about the results of the study. For research to have an impact on practice, policy, law, etc., which is particularly important when it comes to forensic research, the findings must be disseminated widely. Fortunately, there are several common ways to disseminate research results, with the two most common approaches being publications and presentations (see DeMatteo et al., 2020, for a fuller discussion of the various types of publications).

Publications

Publications come in various forms, including peer-reviewed articles, book chapters, books, law review articles, newsletters, trade magazines, and blogs. We briefly discussed some of these outlets in Chapter 2. However, not all these publication formats are treated equally. In the world of academia, peer-reviewed articles carry the most value. Here is a brief description of how peer review works. When a manuscript is submitted to a scientific journal, the editor invites several people with relevant subject matter expertise to review the manuscript. Typically, peer review is masked, which means neither the manuscript author nor the reviewers are aware of the other's identity. The peer-review process, which is considered the gold standard in publishing, is intended to assess the strengths and weaknesses of the manuscript so the editor can make a publication decision. Of note, when outlining criteria for the admissibility of expert evidence in court, the United States Supreme Court highlighted peer-review and publication as a key factor weighing in favor of admission (see *Daubert v. Merrell Dow Pharmaceuticals, Inc.*, 1993). Although there are quite a few journals that publish forensically relevant research, getting peer-reviewed publications can be challenging. The top-tier journals in the forensic psychology field are highly competitive, with rejection rates of 80–85%.

EXAMPLES OF FORENSIC PSYCHOLOGY JOURNALS

- Behavioral Sciences and the Law
- Criminal Justice and Behavior
- International Journal of Forensic Mental Health
- Journal of the American Academy of Psychiatry and the Law
- Journal of Interpersonal Violence
- Law and Human Behavior
- Psychology, Crime and Law
- Psychology, Public Policy, and Law

Presentations

Another common way to disseminate research results is through presentations. As with publications, there are several types of presentations, the most common of which is a presentation at a professional conference. Most professional organizations hold conferences (typically annually). For those who want to present their research at a conference, they submit a proposal, which is reviewed by (typically) several reviewers before the conference organizers make a decision. At most psychology conferences, presentations are either posters, papers, or symposia. Poster presentations involve presenting research on a poster (perhaps 3′ × 5′). This presentation format is often reserved for student presenters. A paper presentation, despite the name, is a brief oral presentation, typically along with PowerPoint slides. A symposium is a group of related presentations that revolve around the same topic. Several professional organizations that focus on forensic psychology hold annual conferences, including the American Psychology-Law Society (Division 41 of the American Psychological Association) and the International Association of Forensic Mental Health Services. Importantly, conference presentations are not the only type of presentation to consider. For example, presenting research results as part of a continuing education workshop for professionals, or perhaps as part of a webinar lecture series, are great ways to share research with students, early-career professionals, and seasoned veterans.

FORENSIC FUN FACT

In the wake of the COVID-19 pandemic, two large forensic mental health webinar series have emerged: [1] the University of New Mexico School of Medicine's *Law and Mental Health Didactic Series* (https://hsc.unm.edu/medicine/departments/psychiatry/divisions/forensic-services/) and [2] McMaster University's *International Forensic Psychiatry Lecture Series* (https://www.forensicpsychiatryinstitute.com/ifpls/). Both host regular webinars on interesting topics in forensic mental health, provided by some of the field's foremost experts.

CHAPTER TAKEAWAYS

The role of research in academia is firmly entrenched. For hundreds of years, faculty members at colleges and universities have been central in conducting research and disseminating study results. Research has the potential to contribute to our understanding of a topic, push the field forward in meaningful ways, generate revenue, and enhance the reputation of the researchers and school. For forensic psychologists, research is an exciting and fulfilling way to influence practice and policy.

Career Profile: Christopher M. King, J.D., Ph.D.

Where Are You Currently Working, and What Position Do You Hold?

I work at Montclair State University, a public university in Northern New Jersey classified as a high research activity doctoral university—i.e., an R2 university. I am currently Associate Professor of Psychology and Director of Clinical Training for the Psychology Department's Ph.D. Program in Clinical Psychology. I started at Montclair immediately after completing my doctoral internship in health service psychology, and I received tenure and promotion along Montclair State's typical timeline.

What Got You Interested in a Career in Working in Research-Oriented Academia?

It was multidetermined: I'll try to summarize some highlights. My mother is a practicing clinical psychologist, so the apple did not fall far from the tree in terms of me being interested in health service psychology generally. Although my mother has a Psy.D., like many, I was drawn to Ph.D. programs in part due to the funding support they typically offer. I attended the J.D./Ph.D. program at Drexel University. I realized early on that the prospect of working as a lawyer did not appeal to me, although my legal training lent me a scholarly niche for legal research and a deeper understanding of the law than is typical. However, over the course of my doctoral training at Drexel, I realized that I had become passionate about research—and if push came to shove, more so than clinical work. I would often look up the authors of articles and books that impressed me as a doctoral student, and while there were some exceptions, most seemed to be working as university professors. My admiration for my own doctoral program mentors certainly also played an influential role, and I continue to try to approximate what they do as professors.

In terms of things I wanted out of a specific job, I knew I wanted to conduct research at least a few days per week. Most forensic psychology topics and populations were and remain interesting to me. During my graduate training, I noticed myself frequently thinking about the possibility of conducting research at my externship (practicum) and internship sites. And indeed, I gathered data for my thesis and dissertation at my first doctoral externship site, a correctional facility. During my internship year, I fairly quickly sensed that working full-time in a service delivery setting, whether primarily as an evaluator or an interventionist, would likely grow stale for me. I also did not resonate with formalities, such as having administrative procedures that needed to be followed to call out sick, and I maintain a preference for casualness to this day! I wondered about the possibility of working primarily as a researcher in some sort of department or unit of a correctional or forensic mental health facility or system, as a few scholars whose research I admired did. However, some cursory browsing around suggested to me that such positions were relatively few and far between. There was also another researcher whose work I admired who was in full-time private practice. But however they were able to be a prolific scholar in that context struck me as exceptional, and I did not think I was poised to be as exceptional.

As for the draw of a professorship at an R2 university specifically, on the one hand, I noticed that I was not familiar with certain things that my "R1 (very high research activity university) bound" peers in my doctoral program seemed to be (e.g., federal doctoral research training fellowships). Such things seemed a bit too formal, involved, competitive, and just overall new to me. (It is worth noting that grants, especially large ones, carry much currency at R2 universities, even if the expectation that one consistently secures them as a professor "or else" is less intense relative to R1 universities.) On the other hand, whereas I attended R1 universities for both my undergraduate and doctoral training, I had a peer in my doctoral program who had attended the opposite as an undergraduate: a small liberal arts college. While they spoke highly of their experience there, I thought that I might not enjoy working at an institution where my primary responsibility each day may well be teaching, and I also wanted to be involved in the training of doctoral students. The idea of a balance between those two polarities resonated with me, which I figured was an R2 university.

What Does an Average Workday Look Like for You in Terms of Duties and Responsibilities?

A fair portion of each of my workdays involves monitoring and responding to many emails about a wide variety of things. For example, as a program administrator, I tend to have to make executive decisions about various things each day and usually also engage in some coordination and other preparatory work for various upcoming things. Also connected to this or other service, mentorship, or advising roles, I tend to have a meeting or two to attend most days with different constituents. Once or twice a week, I also teach for a few hours. For the handful of hours in a given day when there is not an entry on my calendar, I typically work on some research, formal consultation, or clinical supervision tasks. I fit occasional and irregular clinical assessment or treatment work in where I can—often in the evenings or on the weekends.

What Is the Most Rewarding Aspect of Your Work?

I engage in a lot of service activities, including supervising doctoral student therapists in a university-based correctional treatment program I developed. While the amount of service I provide is probably more than most would advise, the idea that "in giving, one receives" does deeply resonate with me, and the appreciation that the assorted benefactors of my service activities have conveyed does make me feel good. Also, professional service is, in my experience, unparalleled as a strategy for networking. Thus, at its best, service has been one of the highlights of my career thus far. Besides that, I generally fit the stereotype of a professor: I enjoy having my head in the clouds, continuously learning and thinking about new things and hanging out in my lab, analyzing data and writing up manuscripts.

What Have Been Some of the Most Challenging Things to Navigate in Your Work?

Time management has been the foremost challenge. At an R2 university, you certainly are expected to be publishing and presenting at conferences each year, but you also tend to be pulled in multiple directions besides research. I have not been particularly thoughtful about how I go about balancing research, teaching, service, and practice responsibilities and interests. The problems that flow from saying yes to every opportunity or request that comes your way do not present immediately; they emerge further down the line. You can eventually find yourself overwhelmed with things you take on in one domain to the detriment of things you need to do (e.g., toward promotion) or enjoy doing in others. The idea to just work longer to get it all done creeps in, but it is a bit of a rat wheel, so this eventually leads to more general problems with work–life balance. Thus, I have had to continuously work on recalibrating so as not to linger in periods of feeling burnt out or unhappy. Basically, problem–solving a lack of balance, including engaging in more self-care. The next biggest challenge has probably been managing so many relationships and personalities in my professional life. I have had to figure out different systems to help prompt, schedule, and structure my participation in all these relationships. I also make heavy use of my clinical training in interpersonal effectiveness skills.

If Someone Wanted to Follow in Your Footsteps, What Advice Would You Give Them?

Regarding my personal journey, I performed well as an undergraduate (I maintained a nearly 4.0 GPA), and I had picked up on that you also need to amass a lot of research experience in addition to other things (e.g., some sort of clinical or other applied experience) to make oneself competitive for admission to a Ph.D. program in heath service psychology. So, my first piece of advice is to learn early about what it takes to get admitted to a scientist-practitioner program and then work hard to make yourself competitive. I highlight the scientist-practitioner model of doctoral training in health service psychology, as this type of program is well poised to make one competitive for an eventual university professorship. Of course, I also would not be where I am at were it not for the support and guidance offered to me by my doctoral program mentors (among other mentorship relationships I developed with other professors). As such, I definitely advise cultivating good mentor relations during doctoral training.

Regarding more generalized advice, cultivate your curiosity, creativity, grit, work ethic, and writing abilities. Seek out multiple student leadership positions—including roles that advance the missions of social justice and equity, diversion, and inclusion. Furthermore, go a good bit beyond that which is minimally required by your program or exhibited by your peers headed toward careers in clinical practice. Try to develop niches as a researcher in terms of skills or areas of inquiry, apply for student grants, and yield presentations and publications each year. Finally, amass some teaching experience, ideally as an instructor of record.

Career Profile: Jenni Cox, Ph.D.

Where Are You Currently Working, and What Position Do You Hold?

I am currently Associate Professor of Clinical Psychology (Psychology–Law track) at the University of Alabama.

What Got You Interested in a Career in Working in Research-Focused Academia?

While an undergraduate, I started working as a research assistant in a professor's lab. I thought I wanted to be in the FBI, and this was the only professor at my small liberal arts college who taught forensic psychology. I was certain working in this lab was my first step to Quantico. Over a year, we did a project on technology and identity development in adolescence. I found every step of the process (except the IRB application) fascinating. I loved reading and talking about ideas. I loved designing the methodology and troubleshooting obstacles. I even loved cleaning and analyzing the data. It was awesome to work through our results and make sense of our findings. In short, it was fun. That year, we won an award for best undergraduate research at the Virginia Psychological Association conference (maybe I peaked early!?). I was hooked.

I love to learn and am intrinsically curious about the human experience. People are inherently messy and complicated. I love that. No matter how much we learn about humanity, there are always more questions. Pursuing a research career essentially allows me to be a lifelong learner of human behavior. I chose to focus my research on the criminal legal system because I believe all of us are more than the worst thing we have ever done. Initially,

I was fascinated by the factors that led "good" people to do "bad" things. Yet I increasingly understood the distinction between "good" and "bad" is nebulous and humans exist in context. Perhaps it is naïve, but I hope a better understanding of the systems and contexts that lead to "bad" behavior can translate into prevention and intervention. Because a substantial portion of my responsibilities include creating and disseminating research, I have the time and space to investigate this nuance.

Although my first love is research, teaching is a close second. I was drawn to research academia because I love teaching and learning from my students. I like the challenge of effectively communicating complex psychological theories and making connections between these theories and our daily lives. The university setting is perhaps the first place where young people are required to engage in critical thinking. In a cultural age where we are all inundated with alternative facts and fake news, helping students become critical thinkers and then challenging students to use these skills is, perhaps, the most meaningful work I can do. (And if I am being completely honest, I am also a fan of wearing jeans, t-shirts, and flip-flops, which are far more acceptable in a university setting than most other workplaces.)

What Does an Average Workday Look Like for You, in Terms of Duties and Responsibilities?

On paper, I am supposed to spend 40% of my week teaching, 40% doing research, and 20% providing service to the university and/or professional field. The more accurate breakdown is 20% teaching, 5% research, 35% service, and 137% meetings.

The activities related to my roles as researcher and mentor significantly overlap. Broadly, my research concerns the intersection of psychology and the criminal legal system. I design and execute studies to understand [1] how people encounter the system and [2] how they progress through the system. All my research is team science; I hate science-ing alone. On any given day, I will meet with research collaborators and/or students to discuss various research projects and determine how to push our work forward. I stay engaged with my community partners, including district attorneys, judges, and mental healthcare providers. These folks are doing incredibly hard and meaningful work, and I am grateful they let me share our science. I meet with graduate students regularly to support their progress through the program. On rare occasions, I find time to write and translate our research into articles for scholarly and practitioner journals.

Much of my "teaching" time is dedicated to supervising graduate student clinical work, and this includes regular supervision meetings and direct observations and interactions with clients. Some semesters I have a traditional classroom-based lecture class. Many semesters I "buyout" of teaching, meaning I use grant funding to "buy" my teaching time and reallocate it to research.

My service activities include serving on committees within the department, college, and university (e.g., departmental clinical training committee, the university's faculty senate). I am actively involved in the American Psychology-Law Society and am fortunate to work with the brightest scholars and clinicians in the field through this organization. I also serve as Associate Editor of *Law and Human Behavior* (AP-LS's official journal) on other journal editorial boards and review research grant applications to help federal agencies (e.g., National Science Foundation, National Institutes of Justice) determine what projects to support.

What Is the Most Rewarding Aspect of Your Work?

Mentoring future scientists, clinicians, and teachers is absolutely my favorite part of my job. I had—and continue to have—the very best mentors who support me professionally and personally. I want to pass this on and create relationships in which my students and mentees feel supported and challenged but also autonomous. I enjoy supporting people as they grow and discover their own interests and talents. I am fortunate that my position allows me to teach and serve as a research mentor at both the undergraduate and graduate levels. Working across this developmental span is challenging in that students present with a range of knowledge and capabilities. As a licensed clinical psychologist, I also provide direct clinical supervision for graduate student trainees in therapy and forensic mental health assessment. There is notable overlap in the competencies needed to be effective in classroom teaching, research mentoring, and clinical supervision. Yet each of these roles also requires unique skills, and I find a lot of joy in working to meet each student where they are at. It is incredibly rewarding to witness students excel and know I played a small role in their journey.

What Have Been Some of the Most Challenging Things to Navigate in Your Work?

There is a toxic "publish or perish" mentality in many academic research spaces. This is the idea that a "successful" academic disseminates their research via top-tier scholarly journals and, in the absence of multiple publications, their work does not have value. The tenure system at many universities was initially put into place to allow academics freedom to conduct riskier science without fear of retribution. In reality, this system fuels the "publish or perish" problem, as promotion is predicated on one's research "productivity."

Early in my career, I bought into this problematic mentality that my worth as a scholar and teacher was directly correlated with the number of lines on my CV. I worked around the clock. I published a lot, said "yes!" to every service opportunity, and agreed to mentor many students. I applied for and was granted tenure and promotion a year early! On the night my husband and I went out to dinner to celebrate, I started our meal by saying, "You know, if I keep at it, I can be promoted to full professor before I turn 40!" He wanted to celebrate our current win. I wanted to keep publishing, for fear that my value as an academic could plummet any day.

I was exhausted. My physical and mental health suffered. Then the global COVID-19 pandemic hit. The small silver lining was that the associated social distancing measures allowed me time and space to reflect on my values as a researcher. My joy comes not from publishing but *working with* and *learning from* people. I love research because I love moving toward a more complete understanding of the human experience. Sure, I appreciate the endorphin hit when I receive notification of an accepted manuscript. But when I am done with this gig, a couple of hundred people will have read my publications. No one (me included) will remember my h-index. I will, however, remember my relationships with my students, colleagues, and community partners.

The allure of the "productivity = worth" myth is strong. I continue to work against this mindset and, instead, focus on the ways in which my job (because at the end of the day, it is just a job) serves my values. I also talk openly with my colleagues and students about how this culture stifles our curiosity and leads to faulty science. I am not particularly optimistic that the "publish or perish" mentality will perish during my professional lifetime. However, I do believe that the more we stop feeding into this toxic mindset, the weaker it will become.

If Someone Wanted to Follow in Your Footsteps, What Advice Would You Give Them?

First, stop watching *Criminal Minds* and start reading. Read anything that could teach you about human behavior because forensic psychology is ultimately the study of human behavior in a specific context. To ask the right questions within the forensic psychology realm, we must have a comprehensive understanding of human behavior across contexts. Second, get involved in the research process. This part can be so hard! I teach at a large institution, and there are many more undergrads interested in my research than I have the ability to take on. If you cannot find someone doing research in the area you ultimately want to pursue, don't sweat it. Get your foot in the door with any research lab and learn everything you can about the research process.

Also, be persistent. Psychology doctoral programs are competitive, and programs with a forensic training focus are even more so. Many factors determine who is accepted into programs, including grades, research and clinical experience, training fit, and luck. Research-focused academic positions are even more competitive, and luck plays an outsized role in who ends up getting the offer. Rejection stinks. More than once, I have wanted to give up. Sometimes, I still want to give up. But in the end, there is absolutely nothing else in the world I would rather do.

REFERENCES

Berryessa, C. M., & Wohlstetter, B. (2019). The psychopathic "label" and effects on punishment outcomes: A meta-analysis. *Law and Human Behavior, 43*(1), 9–25. https://psycnet.apa.org/doi/10.1037/lhb0000317

Creswell, J. W., & Creswell, D. D. (2022). *Research design: Qualitative, quantitative, and mixed methods* (6th ed.). SAGE.

Cuellar, J. (2024, March 27). College vs. university: What's the difference? *Best Colleges.* https://www.bestcolleges.com/blog/difference-between-college-and-university/

Daubert v. Merrell Dow Pharmaceuticals, Inc., 509 U.S. 579 (1993).

DeMatteo, D., Edens, J. F., Galloway, M., Cox, J., Smith, S. T., Koller, J. P., & Bersoff, B. (2014). Investigating the role of the Psychopathy Checklist-Revised in United States case law. *Psychology, Public Policy, and Law, 20*(1), 96–107. https://psycnet.apa.org/doi/10.1037/a0035452

DeMatteo, D., Fairfax-Columbo, J., & Desai, A. (2020). *Becoming a forensic psychologist.* Routledge.

DeMatteo, D., Krauss, D. A., Fishel, S., & Wiltsie, K. (in press). *Forensic mental health practice and the law: A primer for clinicians, researchers, and consultants.* Oxford University Press.

Flack, D., Fishel, S., Wiltsie, K., Kudatzky, A., & DeMatteo, D. (2022). Following up after *Moore & Hall*: A national survey of state legislation defining intellectual disability. *Psychology, Public Policy, and Law, 28*(4), 459–478. https://psycnet.apa.org/doi/10.1037/law0000372

Huss, M. T. (2013). *Forensic psychology: Research, clinical practice, and application* (2nd ed.). Wiley.

Kazdin, A. E. (2021). *Research design in clinical psychology* (5th ed.). Cambridge University Press. https://doi.org/10.1017/9781108993647

Marczyk, G., DeMatteo, D., & Festinger, D. (2005). *Essentials of research design and methodology.* Wiley.

Meaux, L., Cox, J., Edens, J. F., DeMatteo, D., Martinez, A., & Bownes, E. (2022). The Personality Assessment Inventory in U.S. case law: A survey and examination of relevance to legal proceedings. *Journal of Personality Assessment, 104*(2), 179–191. https://doi.org/10.1080/00223891.2021.1975723

Mitchell, O., Wilson, D. B., Eggers, A., & MacKenzie, D. L. (2012). Assessing the effectiveness of drug courts on recidivism: A meta-analytic review of traditional and non-traditional drug courts. *Journal of Criminal Justice, 40*, 60–71. http://dx.doi.org/10.1016/j.jcrimjus.2011.11.009

National Institutes of Health. (n.d.). *About NIH.* https://www.nih.gov/about-nih

National Institute of Justice. (n.d.). *About the National Institute of Justice.* https://nij.ojp.gov/about/about-nij

National Science Foundation. (n.d.). *About NSF.* https://new.nsf.gov/about

Office of Justice Programs. (n.d.). *About us.* https://www.ojp.gov/about

Ogonah, M. G.T., Seyedsalehi, A., Whiting, D., & Fazel, S. (2023). Violence risk assessment instruments in forensic psychiatric populations: A systematic review and meta-analysis. *Lancet Psychiatry, 10,* 780–789. https://doi.org/10.1016/s2215-0366(23)00256-0

Pirelli, G., Beatty, R. A., & Zapf, P. A. (Eds.). (2017). *The ethical practice of forensic psychology: A casebook.* Oxford University Press.

Protection of Human Subjects, 45 C.F.R. § 46. (2009). https://www.hhs.gov/ohrp/sites/default/files/ohrp/policy/ohrpregulations.pdf

Rosenfeld, B., & Penrod, S. D. (Eds.). (2011). *Research methods in forensic psychology.* Wiley.

Ross, K. M., & Durrani, A. (2023, July 7). College vs. university: What's the difference? *U.S. News & World Report.* https://www.usnews.com/education/best-global-universities/articles/college-vs-university-whats-the-difference

Rudolph, F. (1991). *The American college and university: A history* (2nd ed.). University of Georgia Press.

Singh, J. P., Grann, M., & Fazel, S. (2011). A comparative study of violence risk assessment tools: A systematic review and meta regression analysis of 68 studies involving 25,980 participants. *Clinical Psychology Review, 31,* 499–513. https://doi.org/10.1016/j.cpr.2010.11.009

Skeem, J. L., Douglas, K. S., & Lilienfeld, S. O. (Eds.). (2009). *Psychological science in the courtroom: Consensus and controversy.* The Guilford Press.

Substance Abuse and Mental Health Services Administration. (n.d.). *About us.* https://www.samhsa.gov/about-us

Wilson, H. A., & Hoge, R. D. (2013). The effect of youth diversion programs on recidivism: A meta-analytic review. *Criminal Justice and Behavior, 40*(5), 497–518. https://psycnet.apa.org/doi/10.1177/0093854812451089

CHAPTER 5

Practice-Oriented and Teaching-Focused Academia

An Overview of Less Traditional Pathways in Academia for Forensic Psychologists

When many aspiring forensic psychologists visualize academia, they picture the grind and glory of amassing peer-reviewed publications, writing books, seeking grant money, founding research and policy centers, and consulting on important policy matters. Indeed, the grandeur of positions in traditional research academia is appealing! But what exactly are aspiring forensic psychologists to do when they are interested in a career in academia but have little desire to live according to the "publish or perish" mentality? Not to worry—this chapter provides an overview of other academic avenues individuals might pursue. This chapter focuses on opportunities in "professional" academic settings, including Psy.D. programs, medical academia, and legal academia. It also discusses careers in teaching-focused academia.

KNOW THE LINGO

"Publish or perish" refers to the idea that success in publishing is disproportionately weighted in determining academic success (e.g., de Rond & Miller, 2005).

DOCTOR OF PSYCHOLOGY (PSY.D.) PROGRAMS

Doctor of Psychology programs—or Psy.D. programs, for short—are doctoral programs for students who are more interested in providing clinical services than in carrying out research. In Psy.D. programs, training is geared toward the

DOI: 10.4324/9781003408857-7

delivery of evidence-based interventions or the conducting of psychological assessments. Similar to Ph.D. degrees, Psy.D. degrees are available in different subfields, including clinical psychology, counseling psychology, and educational psychology. There is usually substantially less emphasis on conducting empirical research than in a Ph.D. program. However, in an effort to train well-rounded practicing psychologists, many Psy.D. programs require students to complete thesis and dissertation projects (Michalski & Fowler, 2016).

Psy.D. programs sometimes exist in traditional university settings, but they may also exist as independent professional schools. Using Massachusetts as an example, Springfield College in Springfield, MA—a university that hosts both undergraduate and graduate programs spanning myriad disciplines—offers a Psy.D. in Counseling Psychology (www.springfield. edu/). In contrast, William James College—formerly the Massachusetts School of Professional Psychology—is a standalone professional school in Newton, MA, that offers only graduate-level training programs pertaining to behavioral health (https://www.williamjames.edu/). William James College hosts a Psy.D. in Clinical Psychology program; through this program, students can pursue a concentration in forensic psychology.

So how exactly do academia-inclined aspiring forensic psychologists choose whether working in a Psy.D. program is a preferable career path compared to working in a Ph.D. program? We offer several key factors for consideration: (1) graduate training models, (2) job qualifications and expectations, (3) typical student/faculty composition, (4) mentorship obligations, and (5) the availability of specialized psychology and law programs.

Graduate Training Models

Doctoral psychology programs tend to adhere to one of two predominant training models: the Boulder model or the Vail model (Norcross & Castle, 2002). Established at a 1949 psychology training conference in Boulder, CO, the Boulder model emphasizes that equivalent weight need be placed on honing students' clinical skills and their research proficiency. The Boulder model champions clinical psychologists as being scientist-practitioners who can function equally well in practice settings and academic settings. Research-wise, programs following the Boulder model focus on training students to be *producers* of research. Typically, Ph.D. programs in psychology follow this approach.

In contrast, the Vail model originates from a 1973 national psychology training conference held in Vail, CO. Training programs adhering to the Vail model emphasize the practice of psychology. Students at Vail model programs may receive some coursework in research and statistics but with a focus on training *consumers* of research. Vail model programs champion psychologists being clinician-scientists (also known as practitioner-scholars), who use research to inform their clinical practice. The Vail model training ideology is typical of Psy.D. programs.

Job Qualifications and Expectations

Regardless of which type of doctoral academic setting an individual selects, achieving tenure is the predominant metric of success as a faculty member. Generally speaking, tenure reflects excellence in some or all of the domains of research, teaching, and service. Exact proportions vary depending on the type of academic appointment a faculty member has (i.e., clinical, research, or teaching focus), but the underlying formula remains the same (APA Committee on Women in Psychology, 2017).

Understanding the typical qualifications and expectations of faculty members in Psy.D. versus Ph.D. programs is imperative, as it demarcates the relative emphasis placed on clinical practice, research, or teaching that are heavily weighted in awarding tenure. A 2015 survey of job postings for doctoral psychology programs indicated several key differences in the applicant qualifications that Psy.D. programs were looking for as compared to Ph.D. programs (Merced et al., 2015). First, Psy.D. programs appeared more open to individuals from varied training backgrounds (either Psy.D. or Ph.D.), while Ph.D. programs tended to favor a Ph.D. as the required credential. Second, Psy.D. program postings seemed to value clinical experience (being licensed or licensed-eligible) more highly than did Ph.D. programs. Third, Ph.D. program postings weighted publication records more highly. Fourth, to the extent that a specific training model preference was stated, Psy.D. programs tended to emphasize the Vail model while Ph.D. programs tended to emphasize the Boulder model. Notably, both Psy.D. and Ph.D. job postings seemed to place equivalent value on prior teaching experience.

Concerning job expectations and responsibilities, several key differences emerged; some of these differences might be expected based on the aforementioned distinctions between Psy.D. and Ph.D. programs. Psy.D. program job postings were more likely to indicate clinical supervision and advising (as opposed to mentoring) as explicit job responsibilities. In contrast, Ph.D. job postings were more likely to emphasize conducting and publishing research, securing external funding, and mentoring as explicit job responsibilities. Perhaps surprisingly, Psy.D. programs outlined research supervision as an explicit job duty more often than Ph.D. programs did, though this may have reflected the same duty being encompassed in the expectation of faculty in Ph.D. programs to conduct and publish research and provide mentorship. Also surprisingly, Ph.D. programs were more likely to emphasize teaching as a job duty than were Psy.D. programs. Both types of programs placed equal emphasis on departmental service as a job expectation. However, note that the aforementioned describes job expectations broadly. Individual programs may differ in terms of their job emphases.

KNOW THE LINGO

Advising refers to providing students support in completing doctoral program requirements. In contrast, mentors also provide career support and psychosocial support to mentees (Lunsford, 2012).

Typical Student/Faculty Composition

A third prominent factor in determining whether employment at a Psy.D. program or a Ph.D. program is a better fit for your career as a forensic psychologist is the type of students and colleagues with whom you will be working. Regarding the student body, historically, Psy.D. programs are less selective than Ph.D. programs. They often have higher acceptance rates and support larger cohorts (Norcross et al., 2010). Also—as might be expected given that Psy.D. programs have a lesser research emphasis—Psy.D. students publish less frequently during their training than Ph.D. students (Lund et al., 2016). Concerning jobs, Psy.D. students are more likely than Ph.D. students to seek clinical jobs upon graduation, while Ph.D. students may be more likely to seek research and academic jobs. Also, Psy.D. programs generally provide substantially less financial assistance for their students than Ph.D. programs, resulting in higher debt loads upon graduation (Norcross et al., 2018).

Regarding faculty colleagues, Psy.D. programs consist of faculty from a more diverse array of theoretical orientations than Ph.D. programs. For example, research-oriented Ph.D. programs house predominantly faculty from cognitive-behavioral orientations, whereas at Psy.D. programs, individuals are also quite likely to encounter faculty from psychodynamic, behavioral, humanistic, or systems orientations (Norcross et al., 2010, 2018). Further, Psy.D. programs tend to recruit and employ faculty from both Ph.D. and Psy.D. backgrounds, while Ph.D. programs predominantly recruit faculty with a Ph.D. (Merced et al., 2015).

Mentorship Obligations

The expectation to provide close mentorship to doctoral candidates is a fourth important factor in choosing between working at a Psy.D. program or Ph.D. program. Many Ph.D. programs utilize a mentorship model in which students work with an assigned mentor. In this sense, mentorship is a central component of Ph.D. programs. By comparison, Psy.D. programs are significantly less likely to offer extensive mentorship. Further, Psy.D. students are less likely to endorse having found a mentor during their graduate training than are Ph.D. students (Mangione et al., 2018). Several factors characteristic of Psy.D. programs contribute to this, including higher student-teacher ratios, having more part-time faculty, and having shorter average completion times, resulting in less time for students and faculty to engage with each other (Ward et al., 2004).

Availability of Specialized Law-Psychology Programs

A final consideration when choosing between working in a Ph.D. versus a Psy.D. program is the likelihood of working with like-minded individuals with similar interests. In seeking out academic jobs, the availability of positions is always a crucial concern. In recent years, the academic landscape in psychology has shifted drastically, with full-time tenure-track or tenured positions being held by only about 30% of professors (Boysen, 2020). This scarcity makes it competitive to obtain academic jobs in psychology and is only compounded if pursuing a specialty program. Indeed, many academics who specialize in forensic psychology may be the lone representative in their department for that discipline.

However, a handful of doctoral programs offer a specific forensic focus in their graduate training. The American Psychology-Law Society regularly publishes its "Guide to Graduate Programs in Forensic and Legal Psychology" (hereinafter, "Guide"), found on its website. The Guide provides a comprehensive listing of training programs in law and psychology. It includes a listing of doctoral psychology programs that offer some type of forensic or legal psychology emphasis or concentration in their training. As of 2023, the Guide identified over 20 Ph.D. programs with this specialized training focus. In contrast, under 10 Psy.D. programs were identified as having a forensic or legal psychology specialization.

AMERICAN PSYCHOLOGY-LAW SOCIETY

The American Psychology-Law Society is a division of the American Psychological Association (APA Division 41). It is a membership organization for both professionals (social scientists and legal professionals) and students. It focuses on advancing contributions that psychological science makes to the law, promoting education at the intersection of law and psychology, and keeping psychologists and legal professionals apprised of advances in psycholegal research and practice. For more information, visit www.ap-ls.org.

Summary

In summary, though the pathway to tenure is similar in both Psy.D. and Ph.D. programs, the two program types vary substantially in the training ideology they typically employ (Ph.D. Boulder model, Psy.D. Vail model), the types of students and faculty that they attract, the job duties they emphasize, and the level of mentorship that is expected of faculty. Additionally, though many general Ph.D. and Psy.D. programs exist in the United States and Canada, very few emphasize specialized training in psychology and law (e.g., forensic psychology, legal psychology). The programs that do exist are more plentiful in Ph.D. than in Psy.D. settings. Though the aforementioned likely does not represent the full nuance and complexity of the differences between Psy.D. programs and Ph.D. programs, we hope it serves as a good starting point and provides some general guideposts for individuals deciding which path to pursue if they are interested in a career in doctoral academia.

MEDICAL AND LEGAL ACADEMIA

Academic Health Centers

Given that doctoral-level forensic psychologists obtained their training at doctoral psychology programs, it makes intuitive sense that doctoral psychology programs are the assumed setting for academic psychologists to ply their trade. However, medical schools, alternatively known as academic medical centers or academic health centers (AHCs), are an oft-overlooked academic setting in which the skillset of forensic psychologists is highly valued. AHCs represent interprofessional healthcare provision and healthcare education settings. They recruit students and providers from diverse training backgrounds, calling upon their varied areas of expertise to promote interdisciplinary, team-based care.

Psychologists have long taught and practiced in AHC settings, and their representation is steadily growing. In 1955, AHC psychologists numbered under 400; by the mid-2000s, they numbered over 4,000 (Robiner et al., 2014). Though spread across numerous types of medical school departments, most psychologists in AHCs are congregated in departments of psychiatry, psychology, and pediatrics (Robiner et al., 2014). In fact, psychologists are so prevalent in AHCs that the Association of Psychologists in Academic Health Centers (APAHC, www.ahcpsychologists.org) was formed in 1981.

Psychologists make key contributions to AHCs. These contributions include providing psychological services, including therapy and assessment services; participating in grant-funded research; teaching behavioral medicine didactics to residents; supporting medical trainees and medical faculty in research; and helping medical trainees and medical faculty hone their skills in communicating with patients. Additionally, psychologists are uniquely positioned to help promote patient adherence to medical treatments. Further, psychologists may even provide clinical supervision to medical residents in family medicine residencies or psychiatry residencies. Medical schools also increasingly offer pre-doctoral psychology internships, where psychologists serve as core faculty members (see Robiner et al., 2014, 2021). As of 2014, over 100 psychology internships were hosted by or affiliated with a medical school; a full listing can be found on the Association of Psychology Postdoctoral and Internship Centers website (www.appic.org/).

JOB SEARCH STRATEGY

Like the idea of working in an AHC but wondering how to find which ones might most cater to forensic interests? One good search strategy might be seeking out AHCs that host training programs in psychology (pre-doctoral internships and postdoctoral fellowships). You can find regularly updated databases of such training sites on the AP-LS Student Committee website (www.apls-students.org). A second strategy might be seeking out AHCs that host fellowship programs in forensic psychiatry. You can find a regularly updated database of these training sites at the American Academy of Psychiatry and the Law (AAPL) website (www.aapl.org).

Law Schools

A final practitioner-oriented setting in which forensic psychologists may work is a law school. "A law school?" you ask. "How in the world can one practice forensic psychology in a law school?" Indeed, this is a valid question—and sort of a trick question. Though law schools are not focused on churning out forensic psychologists, they do generate practitioners—*legal practitioners*. Legal practitioners interface with other lawyers, judges, clients, and policy professionals. Truly, the craft of a barred attorney hinges on an ability to persuade others.

Calls for greater emphasis on behavioral health literacy and other psychological topics in legal education have long been made (see, e.g., Watson, 1963; Wexler, 1990; Winick & Wexler, 2006). To this end, some law schools offer courses addressing the intersection of behavioral health and the law, such as a mental health law course or a behavioral sciences and the law course. Still other schools offer opportunities for experiential learning, such as having a mental health law clinic.

There are several classic paths to becoming a law professor; all of them involve obtaining a law degree (Leiter, 2022). Therefore, in general, working in a law school might be a more achievable pathway for forensic psychologists with dual degrees (i.e., J.D./Ph.D. or J.D./Psy.D.). To this end, interdisciplinary training may help provide a "leg up" in obtaining a job in legal academia. For example, in a 2015 review of academic job postings—including 120 postings for law school faculty positions—roughly one-third of law postings indicated that interdisciplinary training was a desirable qualification for applicants (Kleynhans & Bornstein, 2015). Further, a 2016 study of new hires in legal academia revealed that 21% had both a J.D. and a Ph.D. (LoPucki, 2016).

FORENSIC FUN FACT

Though employment in legal academia typically requires a law degree, several forensic psychology "mavericks" have worked in legal academia without a law degree. Salient examples include the late Gary B. Melton, as well as John Monahan and Michael J. Saks. In fact, in 1987, these three pioneers in the field authored the article *Psychologists as Law Professors*. We encourage you to read it!

TEACHING-FOCUSED ACADEMIA

Thus far, we have reviewed research academia (see the preceding chapter) and practice-focused academia. The third and final type of academic institution that employs forensic psychologists is teaching-focused academia. This category of academia exists across the broad spectrum of academic institutions, from undergraduate small liberal arts colleges to large public universities. Forensic psychologists in teaching-focused academia play a pivotal role in imparting knowledge and developing the next generation of professionals in the field. Whether you are considering teaching in a specialized forensic psychology program, a generalized psychology department, or moonlighting as an adjunct professor, this section will help you explore the unique challenges and rewards of teaching-focused academia.

Why Teaching?

Before delving into the nitty gritty of what teaching-focused academia entails for a forensic psychologist, it is worth considering what makes these roles appealing in the first place. As an academic focused on teaching, you have the privilege of witnessing those magical "aha!" moments when students experience a breakthrough in their understanding of complex ideas. You will engage in students' academic development, form meaningful connections, and nurture their professional growth. You may even introduce students to the field of forensic psychology, imparting valuable wisdom that will shape their careers. In teaching-focused academia, the opportunities to leave a lasting impact are vast.

Beyond being a rewarding and impactful job, careers in teaching-focused academia benefit from being in a growing area of the workforce. According to the U.S. Bureau of Labor Statistics (2023a), postsecondary teaching positions are projected to increase over the next decade, driven by the number of students seeking higher education. The data estimated 50,900 postsecondary psychology teachers in 2022, with an expected rise of 5%, or 2,700 new jobs, by 2032. This trend is relevant to forensic psychologists who often are housed in psychology departments and may teach courses on forensic topics or more general psychology courses, such as abnormal (clinical) psychology and research methods.

A FIELD ON THE RISE

The rise in teaching positions is indicative of a broader trend within the field of psychology, which is expected to grow substantially over the next decade. Projections indicate a 9% increase of jobs in psychology compared to the average growth rate of 3% for all occupations (Bureau of Labor Statistics, 2023b).

Teaching Professors

The title and specific responsibilities of a teaching professor can differ across institutions. Generally, a teaching professor is a full-time faculty member whose primary role centers around class instruction. These positions may exist on a tenure track, with ranks of assistant professor, associate professor, or full professor. In contrast, nontenure track full-time faculty may hold other titles, such as lecturer or instructor (Ansburg et al., 2022). Note that these titles do vary, and it is advisable to consult the faculty handbook for information on the specific tracks and ranks offered at each institution. Faculty may also have other roles besides teaching, including professional development, mentorship, or university service roles (Rawn & Fox, 2018). The prevalence of faculty teaching positions varies among institutions; in some, most full-time faculty may emphasize teaching, while in others, teaching professors may coexist in a sea of research or clinical faculty (Boysen, 2020).

What Is a Teaching-Focused Institution?

Teaching-focused institutions are those that prioritize teaching over research activity for faculty members. It can be difficult to identify what the institution emphasizes without interviewing faculty at every school. Both research-focused and teaching-focused academia encompass a wide array of schools, ranging from public to private and from large to small. The distinction between them isn't always clear-cut. Further, many schools occupy a middle ground, incorporating a mix of research, clinical work, and teaching.

Schools are often categorized by the degrees they offer rather than how much emphasis they place on teaching. Teaching-focused institutions tend to focus on bachelor's or associate degrees, although they may also have master's programs. The most common framework for categorizing institutions is the Carnegie Classifications of Institutions of Higher Education (n.d.), colloquially called "Carnegie Classifications." The six Basic Classifications include nearly every college, university, and other institution: doctoral universities, master's colleges and universities, baccalaureate colleges, baccalaureate/associate colleges, associate colleges, and special focus institutions. By looking at universities based on classifications, there are a few signs that can show us how much importance the school probably gives teaching versus research.

Doctoral universities award a minimum of 20 research/scholarship doctoral degrees annually or at least 30 professional practice doctoral degrees in at least two programs. Although many full-time faculty at doctoral universities are research-oriented, some full-time roles may be reserved for professors to teach courses with expectations and performance evaluations revolving around their teaching. For example, the University of California (UC) is a research-intensive university system that has full-time positions and tenure-track ranks for lecturing faculty. UC Irvine offers a Master of Legal and Forensic Psychology degree, and several of the UC schools offer forensic-relevant undergraduate courses. The teaching faculty are appointed to one of three ranks: Assistant Teaching Professor, Associate Teaching Professor, or Teaching Professor. The three appointments are like that of research-focused professors. Uniquely, these faculty members are primarily responsible for teaching courses at any level. The faculty have no responsibilities to engage in research and will typically have a heavier course load compared to the research-focused faculty (University of California, Los Angeles, 2022). The advantage of this structure is the clear path for faculty to obtain job security via tenure, opportunities for merit advancement, and the typical benefits of full-time employment (e.g., insurance, retirement, parental leave).

Master's colleges and universities confer at least 50 master's degrees and fewer than 20 doctoral degrees annually. Typically, these institutions maintain a strong focus on undergraduate education. Programs generally place less emphasis on research compared to doctoral universities; however, faculty may still be required to engage in research activities. This category may appeal to those primarily interested in teaching but who wish to maintain some degree of research productivity (Boysen, 2020). For instance, the University of New Haven is a master's university that offers a forensic concentration for undergraduate psychology majors. Faculty within the university emphasize teaching, although they are expected to engage in research and service as well. Tenured and tenure-track faculty are expected to teach 24 credit hours each academic year (i.e., four classes per semester). Faculty can decrease their courseload by meeting specific research output expectations. The forensic concentration for undergraduates means that more forensic-specific undergraduate classes are offered, increasing the opportunity to teach forensic courses. Additionally, undergraduates will have increased knowledge and interest in forensic psychology, making your mentorship more meaningful (University of New Haven, 2021).

Baccalaureate colleges award 50% of degrees or more at the baccalaureate level, and fewer than 50 master's or 20 doctoral degrees are awarded annually. Faculty members are primarily recruited for teaching, although institutions still expect faculty to engage in other responsibilities (described later in this section). Although the balance between these roles may vary from school to school, the primary emphasis of a baccalaureate college is always undergraduate education, making teaching the faculty's central focus. Baccalaureate/associate colleges are where more than 50% of the degrees are associate's level but have at least one baccalaureate degree. These institutions are functionally like baccalaureate colleges when considering how teaching-oriented they are.

Associate's colleges are where the highest degree level at these institutions is an associate's degree. Many of these institutions are community colleges, focusing on inclusive and affordable higher education. As of 2023, there are over 1,000 community colleges in the United States, encompassing over 10 million enrolled students (American Association of Community Colleges, 2023). Nearly all faculty positions at an associate's college are teaching-focused, as they focus entirely on early undergraduate education. The majority have no requirements for research. Most community colleges offer rudimentary psychology courses, and some even have forensic psychology-specific courses. If you want a flexible job that allows you to teach, teach, teach, this may be your ideal path.

Special focus institutions are dedicated to one specific field, such as law schools, medical schools, and faith-related institutions. Within this category, there are institutions that specialize in psychology training. For example, Adler University offers undergraduate, master's, doctorate, and certificate programs, all in the field of psychology. Notably, the university offers a master's (M.A.) in Forensic Mental Health Leadership, equipping graduates to work in various settings within the forensic mental health system and public safety settings, such as within law enforcement, the courts, crisis services, and community correctional settings. The faculty at Adler prioritizes instruction. Teaching faculty are expected to allocate a minimum of 10% of their time to service or research (Adler University, 2018). Although this type of institution may be ideal for those inclined toward teaching, keep in mind that the programs are small, few and far between, and often have a small faculty. Further, it is near impossible to draw generalizations from this category, as the emphasis varies based on the type of institution.

TYPICAL TEACHING LOADS (BY SEMESTER)

- Doctoral university = one to two courses
- Master's university = three to four courses
- Baccalaureate college = four courses
- Community college = five courses
- Special focus institutions = varies

CHAPTER TAKEAWAYS

Practice-oriented academia may represent solid career pathways for individuals who are not interested in the "publish or perish" mentality. For forensic psychologists who are interested in working in a practice-oriented doctoral program, Psy.D. programs may be optimal. Psy.D. programs may particularly appeal to forensic psychologists who adhere to the Vail model of doctoral training, value working with more clinically oriented students, value having faculty peers from varied theoretical orientations, and want more lenient requirements for mentorship. However, fewer specialized forensic psychology programs are available in Psy.D. settings than in Ph.D. settings. AHCs commonly employ psychologists, including forensic psychologists. Interested forensic psychologists may fare best targeting medical schools that host forensic psychology pre-doctoral internship, postdoctoral fellowship, or forensic psychiatry fellowship programs. Law schools are a less common setting in which to find forensic psychologists. Individuals with dual training (e.g., J.D./Ph.D. or J.D./Psy.D.) may be more competitive for legal academia. Teaching academics play a pivotal role in molding the future generation of forensic psychologists through their influence on students both within and beyond the classroom. There are various career tracks within teaching academia that impact the specifics of your job. Recognize the weight of these factors when contemplating your career path, as they wield significant influence on your teaching course load and other job expectations.

Career Profile: Anthony Perillo, Ph.D.

Where Are You Currently Working, and What Position Do You Hold?

Since 2022, I have worked in the Health Sciences Center of the University of New Mexico School of Medicine. I am Associate Professor in the Department of Psychiatry and Behavioral Sciences. My primary role is as Forensic Training Director for our Forensic Psychology Postdoctoral Fellowship, which accounts for about half of my professional time. The other half of my time goes to a combination of conducting my own forensic evaluations, working on forensic research and policy analysis, and other training activities in the School of Medicine (e.g., didactics for psychiatry residents or clinical psychology interns).

What Got You Interested in a Career in Working in Practice-Oriented Academia?

In graduate school, I wavered between wanting a research-heavy or practice-heavy career many times (and I mean many!). I did two years of full-time clinical work after finishing my Ph.D. but realized I did not find a 100% clinical role exciting; after only two years, I already felt in a rut. I missed the university setting, and I missed contributing to and just talking about research. I ultimately landed in a tenure-track faculty position working in a Psy.D. program. I was not specifically targeting this (my spouse is an academic, and honestly, we were looking for any dual academic hire we could both find rewarding), but I enjoyed being back in an academic setting.

For several reasons, that job started falling apart, and my spouse and I looked for other opportunities. At that stage, we wanted to get closer to family; we were tired of fitting our lives around the jobs we wanted and prioritized fitting our jobs around the lives we wanted. I was willing to let go of academia for that. I asked myself what was most important to me in my job and came to the realization that what I found most rewarding was not specifically research, not specifically clinical work, and not specifically teaching (which I discovered I loved). What drove me was collaboration and mentorship! I loved helping people learn, refine their skills, develop their clinical skills, and find their paths.

When a forensic academic medical center position popped up in my searches near family, I discovered it hit everything I would find rewarding but would also maintain excitement! I enjoy clinical work but do not enjoy a full caseload. I enjoy research but not the pressure to publish. I enjoy teaching but not the lesson planning. In an academic medical center, I have found the balance of clinical work, scholarship, and mentorship/collaboration that works for a "scientist-practitioner" like myself. Our clinical practice drives research initiatives, and the research directly improves clinical practice. The research is very collaborative, both with faculty and with agencies to make a direct impact on policy and our community. Combine that with working with psychology and psychiatry trainees looking to bolster their forensic skills, and I find practice-oriented academia a great fit for clinically minded scientists who want to serve their community.

What Does an Average Workday Look Like for You, in Terms of Duties and Responsibilities?

Most of my Wednesdays and Thursdays are spent in clinical activities: observing trainee evaluations, conducting my own evaluations, and report writing/reviewing. Tuesdays are supervision days, where I have individual and group supervision with fellows, lead the University of New Mexico's Law and Mental Health Series (even though this didactic series is free to the public and offers free continuing education units, it is our fellowship's didactic presentation series; we just open it to the world!), and teach the occasional psychiatry didactic. Mondays I set for policy work and additional evaluations as they come up. Fridays are more of a flex day for me, where I fit the other tasks to be done for the week. That being said, my primary duty is to my postdoctoral fellows, so I prioritize their training and consultation needs whenever possible. *That* being said, my evenings are highly valued and protected for personal time (young child at home). I have found for those days where a traditional 9-to-5 won't cut it for hypersensitive deadlines, bumping emails and more low-effort administrative tasks until after the child goes to bed gives me time to maximize the workday for more mentally intensive tasks.

What Is the Most Rewarding Aspect of Your Work?

Many people contemplating clinical versus research careers face the struggle of where they want to make their impact: the clinical path, where you directly see your impact with a small subset of people or a research path, where you can potentially make a wider impact but are less likely to directly "see" it. Being a forensic psychologist in an academic medical center is the best of both worlds! I'm simultaneously asked to serve my community by providing forensic evaluations and to use my research skills to address immediate and long-term issues in our state's legal and mental health systems. To top it off, my favorite part of academia was working with students. Being a training director allows me to continue mentorship and collaborate with trainees as we impact our field and policy together.

What Have Been Some of the Most Challenging Things to Navigate in Your Work?

For academic faculty positions broadly, the "soft money" label (positions funded by outside contracts rather than directly by the institution) can be daunting as you get situated. I have found a clinical soft money position not as stressful in that regard (though to be fair, the training director portion of my salary is actually set and supported by the state), but I have had to adjust to being more mindful of my work hours and output to demonstrate that I am indeed supporting my position through the evaluations I do and grants that fund my time. Specifically as a training director, my biggest challenge in mentoring fellows is consulting as they refine their forensic report writing. At times, it can be challenging to encourage fellows' agency to try new organizational styles, different framings, different ways of presenting data, etc., and mesh that with the conventions of the parties that will read these reports. Certain judges and attorneys can expect or otherwise prefer to see specific phrasing or placement. I want fellows to develop into their own forensic psychologist but simultaneously want to prepare them to succeed through immediate impact.

If Someone Wanted to Follow in Your Footsteps, What Advice Would You Give Them?

I always encourage people to take a step back and ask a very basic question: Why? Why do you want to follow this track? Your answer might help prioritize which aspects of the job are most important to you or even open doors to related jobs. Beyond that, like with many jobs, talking with people doing the work you see for yourself goes a long way. If you are in graduate school, doing practica in medical settings where you work with faculty can open those doors. In terms of active pursuit of jobs, again, network, but even more so, inquire directly with people in Schools of Medicine doing the kind of work that interests you! Academic medical center positions are generally "soft money" positions, meaning the person funds their salary through the clinical services they provide and funding they have from grants. This also means, in contrast with traditional faculty positions, there are often easier pathways for opening hiring lines (since medical faculty will end up largely funding the position created).

Career Profile: Cassie Bailey, Ph.D.

Where Are You Currently Working, and What Position Do You Hold?

I currently work as Tenure-Track Assistant Professor of Clinical Psychology at Metropolitan State University of Denver (MSU of Denver). At MSU of

Denver, I have taught Abnormal Psychology, Forensic Psychology, Psychology of Violence and Aggression, Statistics for the Social and Behavioral Sciences, Introduction to Psychology, and a study abroad course in Mexico. I also have an active research lab (i.e., the Research for Justice Psychology Lab), where my students and I broadly research topics related to Latinx mental health disparities, Spanish language, and forensic assessment. Part of my job as a professor also includes service responsibilities. I am currently Assistant Chair of the Institutional Review Board for my university, Chair of the Student Award Committee for my department, Chair of the Clinical/Forensic Undocumented Special Interest Group Collaborative of the National Latinx Psychological Association, and Secretary and Division 41 Representative of the American Psychological Association's Divisions of Social Justice.

In my free time, I run my private practice (i.e., Bailey Bilingual Forensic Psychology, LLC), where I conduct court-ordered and privately retained forensic evaluations (e.g., competence to stand trial, criminal responsibility, juvenile reverse transfer, immigration evaluations) in English and Spanish.

What Got You Interested in a Career in Working in Teaching-Focused Academia?

I love doing research but noticed my intrinsic motivation for conducting research started waning when it was a requirement I had to fulfill rather than a hobby I got to do. Working in teaching-focused academia, I am able to do research at my own pace, without the pressure of meeting the metrics of a Carnegie-classified (e.g., R1) research institution. I also found teaching quite enjoyable as a graduate student and wanted to pursue that passion further. One of the reasons I find teaching enjoyable is that it forces you to stay up to date on the newest research and literature, and you can learn fresh perspectives from people (i.e., students) whose voices are not usually represented in the research literature beyond that of a research subject. Another reason I chose a teaching-focused position in academia is that it provides me with the flexibility to take private practice cases, particularly during the summer months when I am off-contract (i.e., not expected to work).

What Does an Average Workday Look Like for You, in Terms of Duties and Responsibilities?

At MSU of Denver, a typical workday includes preparing for class (e.g., reminding myself of the day's lecture), lecturing for one to two courses, holding office/advising hours, attending meetings, grading student assignments, and answering emails. I also set aside one day a week to work specifically on research for at least three hours. Although I am on a 4/4 (i.e.,

I teach four classes each semester), my course load changes depending on various factors, as there are many ways in which you can obtain a course release to lighten your teaching load. Depending on my course load for the semester, I usually have one to two days of "free" time in which I do not have to be at school and have no scheduled responsibilities for my teaching job; on these days, I will work on research or my private practice, which usually consists of meeting with attorneys, reviewing records, evaluating a defendant, administering tests, scoring/interpreting assessment measures, conducting collateral interviews, report writing, or attending trainings (e.g., to familiarize myself with the hottest new assessment measure to hit the market or obtain continuing education credits to maintain my licensure). I also supervise graduate students at the University of Denver both in conducting evaluations and providing outpatient competency restoration treatment.

What Is the Most Rewarding Aspect of Your Work?

Although it is cool when a research article gets accepted for publication, my favorite aspect of my work is "converting" non-psychology majors into prospective psychologists. Specifically, I feel honored when a student reaches out to me to tell me that they have decided to pursue a career in forensic psychology after taking several of my courses. This love and excitement for the field of forensics reminds me of the love and excitement that brought me into the field years ago. This love and excitement are particularly salient when I take students to the American Psychology-Law Society's (American Psychological Association Division 41) annual convention each year, which is usually the students' first research conference. Watching them present and receive kudos from others in the field is especially fulfilling.

What Have Been Some of the Most Challenging Things to Navigate in Your Work?

Teaching-focused academic positions are some of the lowest-paying positions in academia (i.e., in comparison to their rank-equivalent counterparts at other universities). For example, I was able to bring in my yearly teaching salary in six months working one to two private practice cases a month. Further, in addition to the increased teaching workload (many research-focused institutions are on a 2/2 or less), teaching-focused academic positions often do not have the research funding or resources needed to maintain an active research program. This means seeking external funding. However, even when external funding is obtained, the university may not have the appropriate infrastructure to manage the grant, which often means a lot of administrative work and emails for the principal investigator.

If Someone Wanted to Follow in Your Footsteps, What Advice Would You Give Them?

I would recommend beginning by getting acquainted with your undergraduate professors. First, you will need letters of recommendation when applying for graduate school. Second, learning about your professors can open the door to potential teaching and research opportunities, such as working in their research lab, collaborating on a research project, or becoming their teaching assistant. Getting involved in research and teaching early may elucidate whether a career in academia is right for you; even at a teaching university, I still have research requirements for tenure.

I would also recommend taking advantage of any internship opportunities that exist with clinical/forensic populations. Shadowing clinical professionals, working as a probation officer, moonlighting as a security officer for a juvenile detention facility, any contact with the system can help expose you to the field of forensic psychology and better prepare you for graduate school (or help you realize that forensic psychology is not the field for you). Finally, once in graduate school, take opportunities to teach undergraduate students at your university if offered the chance. Additionally, many universities offer trainings/programs to enhance faculty/staff's teaching abilities and are often open to graduate student lecturers as well. Overall, it may be helpful to test the waters and try out different aspects of your desired career before diving in headfirst. Luckily for me, I figured out before studying for the MCAT and getting into medical school that becoming an obstetrician/gynecologist was not the right career path for me.

REFERENCES

Adler University. (2018). *Faculty handbook: Chicago campus.* https://publicdocs.adler.edu/LMS/HLC/Chicago_Campus_Faculty_Handbook.pdf

American Association of Community Colleges. (2023). *Fast facts.* https://www.aacc.nche.edu/research-trends/fast-facts/

American Psychological Association CEMRRAT2 Task Force and Committee on Women in Psychology. (2017). *Surviving and thriving in academia: A guide for members of marginalized groups.* http://www.apa.org/pi/oema/resources/brochures/surviving.aspx

Ansburg, P. I., Basham, M. E., & Gurung, R. A. R. (2022). *Thriving in academia: Building a career at a teaching-focused institution.* American Psychological Association. https://doi.org/10.1037/0000261-000

Boysen, G. A. (2020). *Becoming a psychology professor: Your guide to landing the right academic job.* American Psychological Association. https://doi.org/10.1037/0000152-000

Bureau of Labor Statistics, U.S. Department of Labor. (2023a). *Occupational outlook handbook, postsecondary teachers.* https://www.bls.gov/ooh/education-training-and-library/postsecondary-teachers.htm

Bureau of Labor Statistics, U.S. Department of Labor. (2023b). *Occupational outlook handbook, psychologists.* https://www.bls.gov/ooh/life-physical-and-social-science/psychologists.htm

The Carnegie Classification of Institutions of Higher Education. (n.d.). *Basic classification*. https://carnegieclassifications.acenet.edu/

de Rond, M., & Miller, A. N. (2005). Publish or perish: Bane or boon of academic life? *Journal of Management Inquiry*, *14*(4), 321–329. https://doi.org/10.1177/105649260527685

Kleynhans, A., & Bornstein, B. H. (2015). The competitive advantage of interdisciplinary training in law and social sciences. *AP-LS News, Fall Issue*, 7–10. https://www.apadivisions.org/division-41/publications/newsletters/news/2015/10/issue.pdf

Leiter, B. (2022, November). Paths to law teaching. *The University of Chicago: The Law School*. https://www.law.uchicago.edu/careerservices/pathstolawteaching

LoPucki, L. (2016). Dawn of the discipline-based law faculty. *Journal of Legal Education*, *65*(3), 506–542. https://scholarship.law.ufl.edu/facultypub/1100/

Lund, E. M., Bouchard, L. M., & Thomas, K. B. (2016). Publication productivity of professional psychology internship applicants: An in-depth analysis of APPIC survey data. *Training and Education in Professional Psychology*, *10*(1), 54–60. https://doi.org/10.1037/tep0000105

Lunsford, L. G. (2012). Doctoral advising or mentoring? Effect on student outcomes. *Mentoring & Tutoring" Partnership and Learning*, *20*(2), 251–270. https://doi.org/10.108 0/13611267.2012.678974

Mangione, L., Borden, K. A., Nadkarni, L., Evarts, K., & Hyde, K. (2018). Mentoring in clinical psychology programs: Broadening and deepening. *Training and Education in Professional Psychology*, *12*(1), 4–13. http://dx.doi.org/10.1037/tep0000167

Melton, G. B., Monahan, J., & Saks, M. J. (1987). Psychologists as law professors. *American Psychologist*, *42*(5), 502–509. https://doi.org/10.1037/0003-066X.42.5.502

Merced, M., Stutman, Z., & Mann, S. T. (2015). A developmental lag in the evolution of doctor of psychology programs. *Training and Education in Professional Psychology*, *9*(3), 248–257.

Michalski, D. S., & Fowler, G. (2016, January). Doctoral degrees in psychology: How are they different, or not so different? American Psychological Association. https://www.apa.org/ed/precollege/psn/2016/01/doctoral-degrees

Norcross, J. C., & Castle, P. H. (2002). Appreciating the PsyD: The facts. *Eye on Psi Chi*, *7*(1), 22–26. http://dx.doi.org/10.24839/1092-0803.Eye7.1.22

Norcross, J. C., Ellis, J. L., & Sayette, M. A. (2010). Getting in and getting money: A comparative analysis of admission standards, acceptance rates, and financial assistance across the research-practice continuum in clinical psychology programs. *Training and Education in Professional Psychology*, *4*(2), 99–104. https://doi.org/10.1037/a0014880

Norcross, J. C., Sayette, M. A., & Pomerantz, A. M. (2018). Doctoral training in clinical psychology across 23 years: Continuity and change. *Journal of Clinical Psychology*, *74*, 385–397. https://doi.org/10.1002/jclp.22517

Rawn, C. D., & Fox, J. A. (2018). Understanding the work and perceptions of teaching focused faculty in a changing academic landscape. *Research in Higher Education*, *59*, 591–622. https://doi.org/10.1007/s11162-017-9479-6

Robiner, W. N., Dixon, K. E., Miner, J. L., & Hong, B. A. (2014). Psychologists in medical schools and academic medical centers: Over 100 years of growth, influence, and partnerships. *American Psychologist*, *69*(3), 230–248. https://doi.org/10.1037/a0035472

Robiner, W. N., Hong, B. A., & Ward, W. (2021). Psychologists' contributions to medical education and interprofessional education in medical schools. *Journal of Clinical Psychology in Medical Settings*, *28*, 666–678. https://doi.org/10.1007/s10880-020-09730-8

University of California, Los Angeles. (2022). *Lecturer with security of employment (LSOE) series*. https://apo.ucla.edu/policies-forms/the-call/lecturer-series#I

University of New Haven. (2021). *Governance documents of the University of New Haven*. https://facultysupport.newhaven.edu/wp-content/uploads/2021/08/Governance-Documents-of-the-University-of-New-Haven-8-16-21.pdf

Ward, Y. L., Johnson, W. B., & Campbell, C. D. (2004). Practitioner research vertical teams: A model for mentoring in practitioner-focused doctoral programs. *The Clinical Supervisor, 23*(1), 179–190. https://doi.org/10.1300/J001v23n01_11

Watson, A. S. (1963). Teaching mental health concepts in the law school. *American Journal of Orthopsychiatry, 33*(1), 115–122. http://dx.doi.org/10.1111/j.1939-0025.1963.tb00365.x

Wexler, D. B. (1990). Training in law and behavioral sciences: Issues from a legal educator's perspective. *Behavioral Sciences and the Law, 8*(3), 197–204. http://dx.doi.org/10.1002/bsl.2370080303

Winick, B. J., & Wexler, D. B. (2006). The use of therapeutic jurisprudence in law school clinical education: Transforming the criminal law clinic. *Clinical Law Review, 13*, 605–632.

Part III

Working With Individuals

An Exploration of Clinically Focused Jobs

CHAPTER 6

I Want to Serve the Public!

An Overview of Public Sector Clinical Practice

The intersection between mental health conditions and criminal justice involvement has moved sharply into societal consciousness, and the need for a strong public forensic mental health system has perhaps never been more apparent (see Heilbrun & DeMatteo, in press). Numerous issues involving the overlap between mental health and the criminal justice system currently pose significant policy challenges in the United States. Salient examples include the following:

- The overrepresentation of individuals with mental illness under criminal justice supervision, both in carceral settings and in the community (probation/parole). Many attribute this to inadequate investment in community mental health infrastructure in the wake of deinstitutionalization (Lamb & Weinberger, 2020).
- Concerns over carceral settings (jails and prisons)—such as the Los Angeles County Jail (Cooper, 2013) or Chicago's Cook County Jail (Kuehn, 2014)—becoming de facto mental health treatment centers. This is occurring despite concerns that carceral settings are not optimal for meeting the treatment needs of those with mental health conditions (e.g., Reingle Gonzalez & Connell, 2014; Segal et al., 2018).
- The Opioid Epidemic, which has greatly impacted justice-involved populations (e.g., Scott et al., 2021). This has promoted calls for greater embracing of harm reduction strategies in America (e.g., Yeo et al., 2022).
- The exponential increase in demand for evaluation and treatment services related to adjudicative competency. The shortages in available services to

DOI: 10.4324/9781003408857-9

meet this increased demand is referred to as the Competency Services Crisis (e.g., Gowensmith, 2019).

- Increasing recognition that shortfalls in social determinants of health put individuals at increased risk for *both* mental health challenges and juvenile/criminal justice system involvement. This indicates that decriminalizing mental illness also requires addressing social determinants of health deficits (e.g., Rotter & Compton, 2022).
- Police use of force against individuals with mental illnesses, such as the tragic killing of 27-year-old Walter Wallace, Jr., in Philadelphia in 2020 (e.g., Rushing et al., 2020).
- Police officer wellness and its connection to officer performance (e.g., Mumford et al., 2024).

If any of these issues seem patently unjust and make you "fired up," you may find a forensic mental health career in public service to be appealing. To this end, psychologists have a long history of public service—in fact, the American Psychological Association even has a division devoted to it! Regarding forensic mental health specifically, recent psychologist contributions have been varied and plentiful. For example, psychologists have recently been at the forefront of incorporating telehealth into forensic settings, even before the onset of the COVID-19 pandemic (e.g., Luxton & Niemi, 2020; Manguno-Mire et al., 2007). Additionally, psychologists have worked extensively to examine how police officer wellness connects to job performance (e.g., Panza et al., 2024), as well as to improve police officer interactions with individuals with mental illness (e.g., Crisanti et al., 2022). Further, psychologists have explored various ways to mitigate the Competency Services Crisis by evolving forensic evaluation practices (e.g., Murrie et al., 2023); expanding treatment services, such as outpatient or jail-based restoration (e.g., Gowensmith et al., 2016); and advocating for greater adoption of public health approaches to this issue (e.g., Kois et al., 2023; Pinals & Callahan, 2020).

PSYCHOLOGISTS IN PUBLIC SERVICE

APA Division 18 is comprised of six specialty sections: [1] community and state hospitals, [2] criminal justice, [3] police and public safety, [4] serious mental illness, [5] veterans affairs, and [6] students. It hosts regular webinars, publishes a quarterly journal (*Psychological Services*), and publishes the *Public Service Psychology* newsletter three times per year. Additionally, both the Veterans Affairs and Criminal Justice sections publish regular newsletters. For more information, visit www.publicservicepsych.org/.

An exhaustive review of *all* the ways that forensic psychologists can work in public service is beyond the scope of this chapter. Rather, this chapter seeks to provide food-for-thought for forensic psychologists pondering clinical practice in the public service. First, we will provide a brief review of the sequential intercept model, the predominant model the field of forensic psychology has for addressing the overlap between mental illness and the criminal justice system. We will also briefly explore where psychologists might provide support for various interventions across the sequential intercept model. Second, we will describe four common public mental health settings that may be of interest to forensic psychologists. Third, we will review potential supplemental opportunities for teaching/mentorship and research that may present in these settings. Fourth, we will discuss some of the rewarding and not-so-rewarding aspects of a career in public service. Last, we will review job search strategies that might be helpful in identifying public service career opportunities.

THE SEQUENTIAL INTERCEPT MODEL

As mentioned earlier, the sequential intercept model (SIM; Abreu et al., 2017; Munetz & Griffin, 2006) is the field of forensic mental health's predominant model for remedying the overrepresentation of individuals with mental health challenges in the criminal justice system. The SIM is predicated on the idea that there are six "Intercepts" where individuals who are either involved with or at risk of becoming involved with the criminal justice system can be connected to needed mental health and social support services to prevent recurrent/perpetual justice system involvement.

STAY IN SCHOOL!

It is difficult to do justice (pun intended?) to the nuance and complexity of the SIM in just a few paragraphs. For readers interested in learning more about the SIM, we encourage consultation of either of two great compendium books: *The Sequential Intercept Model and Criminal Justice* (Griffin et al., 2015; updated edition forthcoming) or *Forensic Mental Health: Framing Integrated Solutions* (2nd ed.) (Bratina, 2023).

A summary of each Intercept, its general focus, and example interventions/resources is provided in the following table:

Intercept	General Focus	Example Interventions/ Resources
0 Community Services	Preventing escalation of mental health symptoms to the point where a public safety response may be necessary.	Community Mental Health Centers Crisis Lines Crisis Stabilization Units Mobile Crisis Teams
1 Law Enforcement	Deflection, meaning diversion from arrest and formal criminal justice involvement.	Crisis Intervention Team Training Law Enforcement Assisted Diversion Co-Responder Teams
2 Initial Detention/ Initial Court Hearings	Diversion from formal prosecution.	Community Courts Pretrial Diversion Programs Specialized Pretrial Supervision Rosters Screening for Mental Health Needs
3 Jails/Courts	Diversion from punishment and jail-based assessment and treatment.	Mental Health Courts Drug Courts Veterans Courts Therapeutic Communities Jail Mental Health Services Medication Assisted Treatment
4 Reentry	Reentry planning and reintegration into the community upon return from carceral settings.	Reentry Planning Reentry Courts Warm Handoffs to Community Services
5 Community Corrections	Supporting individuals on community supervision to promote community stabilization and prevent violation of probation/parole.	Specialized Probation Supervision Specialized Parole Supervision Training for Probation/Parole Officers

The SIM represents a systems-based approach to decriminalizing mental illness; in other words, it helps to promote collaboration among key behavioral health and justice system stakeholders. To this end, efforts to help counties to engage in SIM "mapping"—an activity that involves identifying existing resources at each Intercept, as well as exposing gaps that need to be addressed—are generally well-received (Bonfine & Nadler, 2019). Additionally, the Intercepts in the SIM all work in tandem, acting as a series of filters to prevent further penetration into the criminal justice system. To this end, research (Swanson et al., 2023) suggests that counties that invest in interventions at Intercepts 0 and 1 (pre-booking Intercepts) evidence decreases in the number of individuals with a serious mental illness who are booked into county jails. Similarly, counties that invest in interventions at Intercepts 2–5 (post-booking Intercepts) demonstrate increased connection of detained individuals with serious mental illnesses to treatment services.

Forensic psychologists can play key roles at each Intercept. Most SIM interventions involve training legal partners to be more mental health literate or involve direct provision of assessment and treatment services. Therefore, psychologists may consider working for organizations that provide training to justice system stakeholders. They also might consider working for healthcare agencies that staff various SIM interventions. As such interventions typically serve individuals who may not have access to private sector behavioral healthcare (i.e., receive healthcare through the government as opposed to via private insurance), healthcare agencies that staff interventions across the SIM are often run by the government, a public university, or by a non-profit organization. For example, in the City of Albuquerque, New Mexico, two crisis stabilization units currently exist (Intercept 0 interventions). One of these units is run by the Bernalillo County government (www.bernco.gov/department-behavioral-health-services/campus-services/crisis-stabilization-unit/), while the other is run by the University of New Mexico Health System (a non-profit organization affiliated with a public university) (www.unmhealth.org/services/behavioral-health/crisis-triage-center.html). Staying with New Mexico as an example, the University of New Mexico also provides support to justice partners from Intercepts 2 through 5 via various programs, such as the Crisis Intervention Team Extension for Community Healthcare Outcomes (CIT ECHO) program (http://www.gocit.org/cit-knowledge-network.html) and UNM Jail Diversion Services (www.unmhealth.org/services/behavioral-health/jail-diversion-services.html), both affiliated with the UNM Department of Psychiatry and Behavioral Sciences (www.hsc.unm.edu/medicine/departments/psychiatry/).

EXAMPLE ORGANIZATIONS THAT PROVIDE MENTAL HEALTH TRAININGS TO PUBLIC SECTOR AGENCIES OR TO THE PUBLIC

CIT International
(https://www.citinternational.org/)
Council of State Governments Justice Center
(https://csgjusticecenter.org/)
Mental Health First Aid USA
(https://www.mentalhealthfirstaid.org/)
Policy Research Associates
(https://www.prainc.com/)

As another thought, Intercept 0 was designed to better actualize the SIM's Ultimate Intercept: an accessible public mental health system. To this end, psychologists can support the SIM, even when they are not working directly in a forensic setting. For example, psychologists wishing to extend community access to high-quality mental health services may choose to work at county health systems, in Federally Qualified Health Centers, or in Veterans Affairs Health Centers. All these settings serve disadvantaged or specialized populations who may be at greater risk for criminal justice involvement for myriad reasons, ranging from social determinants of health deficits to combat exposure.

COMMON PUBLIC MENTAL HEALTH SETTINGS OF INTEREST TO FORENSIC PSYCHOLOGISTS

Earlier, we reviewed the SIM to provide an example of what building a public forensic mental health system encompasses and the key roles psychologists can play in that system. Next, we will review some common public sector settings that clinical-forensic psychologists might seek employment in: [1] public psychiatric hospitals, [2] public safety settings, [3] forensic mental health services, and [4] carceral settings.

Public Psychiatric Hospitals

Public psychiatric hospitals are inpatient psychiatric facilities that are overseen by the government. Their purpose is to provide both acute and long-term care for individuals with serious mental illnesses (Osborn, 2009). Some patients are quickly stabilized and discharged to less restrictive levels of care in the community; other patients may have more chronic and difficult-to-treat issues, resulting in longer stays. Traditionally, public psychiatric hospitals have employed a medical model in which symptoms are treated with the goal of curing them (and often with psychiatric medication as the first-line intervention). However, given the difficulty of treating some chronically mentally ill patients to symptom remission, public psychiatric hospitals are increasingly embracing the recovery model (Osborn, 2009). This model has less focus on curing symptoms and greater focus on mitigating symptom interference and promoting patient autonomy.

Individuals can be admitted to public psychiatric hospitals either voluntarily or involuntarily (via civil commitment). In recent decades, however, there has been a drastic increase in the number of individuals who are committed to public psychiatric hospitals and who are facing criminal charges (Wik et al., 2020). Such commitments typically have the purpose of evaluating or restoring an individual's adjudicative competence, evaluating their criminal responsibility (e.g., insanity), or to treat them following an insanity adjudication. However, the biggest driver of this increase is accounted for by individuals in need of adjudicative competence services. To this end, Kois and colleagues (2024) estimate that roughly 140,000 adjudicative competence evaluations are ordered every year, with most adjudicative competence evaluations occurring in public psychiatric hospitals (e.g., Gowensmith, 2019).

CASE LAW REVIEW

For an individual to be civilly committed to a public psychiatric hospital due to symptoms of mental illness, the United States Supreme Court has held that the person must pose a danger to themselves or others (*O'Connor v. Donaldson*, 1975). Such potential danger must be proven by clear and convincing evidence (*Addington v. Texas*, 1979).

Psychologists who opt to work in public psychiatric hospitals generally either provide forensic evaluation services or forensic treatment services, though at some facilities, psychologists may do a mix of both. Common forensic evaluation contexts in public psychiatric hospitals are adjudicative competence, civil commitment, mental state at the time of the offense, violence risk assessment, and sentencing considerations. Common forensic treatments provided in public psychiatric hospitals includes competency restoration therapy and risk reduction intervention (i.e., reducing risk of similar incidents happening upon return to the community). Such treatment is often provided in group settings, though it may also be provided individually. Forensic psychologists may also engage in more generalized therapeutic interventions for individuals with serious mental illness.

Public Safety Settings

A growing specialty area in the practice of psychology is that of police and public safety psychology. In fact, psychologists can become board-certified in police and public safety by the American Board of Professional Psychology (www.abpp.org). Per the American Psychological Association, this field is "concerned with assisting law enforcement and other public safety personnel and agencies in carrying out their missions and societal functions with effectiveness, safety, health, and conformity to laws and ethics" (American Psychological Association, 2022). Psychologists who practice in police and public safety settings may be embedded directly in a law enforcement agency, or they may work in a private or group practice and contract services out to public safety agencies. Common activities of police and public safety psychologists include providing screening and therapy services to officers or debriefing officers after a critical incident; completing evaluations, such as pre-employment evaluations or fitness for duty evaluations; providing operational support to law enforcement officers, such as helping in crisis negotiations and/or de-escalation efforts; or providing organizational consultation (e.g., providing trainings, helping to analyze and interpret data, program development and evaluation, consultation on best practices) (Lee, 2024; Monfared, 2022).

SOCIETY FOR POLICE AND CRIMINAL PSYCHOLOGY

The Society for Police and Criminal Psychology is a multidisciplinary professional organization that supports the application of psychology to criminal justice issues. It holds an annual conference, publishes the *Journal of Police and Criminal Psychology* on a quarterly basis, and certifies a Diplomate in Police Psychology. For more information, visit https://www.policepsychology.org/About_SPCP.

KNOW THE LINGO

Pre-employment evaluations for police—also referred to as *suitability* evaluations—are concerned with ensuring that an individual who seeks to become a police officer "possess[es] or demonstrate[es] the requisite psychological traits and characteristics to be a police officer" (Corey & Zelig, 2020, p. xix). In contrast, *fitness for duty* evaluations are concerned with whether a currently-employed officer is "free of an emotional or mental condition that limits [their] ability to perform the essential functions of the job or poses a direct threat to the health or safety of the officer or others" (Corey & Zelig, 2020, p. xix).

Forensic Mental Health Services

In describing forensic mental health services, Melton et al. (2018) identify four distinct models: [1] "institution-based, inpatient model," [2] "institution-based, outpatient model," [3] "community-based, outpatient clinic model," and [4] "community-based, private practitioner model" (pp. 102–103). The former two models both operate out of public psychiatric hospital settings, discussed earlier. The last model—though it involves contracting with a government agency—operates out of a private practice model. In essence, private practitioners become vendors for courts/local governments, and the career setting is a private practice setting. Therefore, we will discuss only the third model here. In this model, a local agency (government-run or contracted to a provider agency) provides outpatient clinical services (though it may be better to say "mobile" clinical services) to specific catchment areas.

Forensic mental health services share a common theme of answering psycholegal questions for courts within a specific catchment area, but otherwise, their setup may vary substantially. For instance, some services may only serve one county, while other services may span an entire state. Additionally, some services may only engage in forensic mental evaluation, while others also provide forensic mental health treatment services (such as competency restoration services). For example, the Georgia Department of Behavioral Health and Development Disabilities' Office of Forensic Services operates statewide, providing evaluation and treatment services regarding both adjudicative competence and criminal responsibility (www.dbhdd.georgia. gov/forensic-services). In contrast, Massachusetts utilizes court clinics to provide more localized evaluation services related to adjudicative competence, criminal responsibility, and civil commitment (both due to mental illnesses and substance use disorders) on more localized levels (www.mass. gov/info-details/forensic-services#court-clinics-).

Carceral Settings

The final common public sector setting we will discuss is carceral settings, meaning county, state, and federal jails and prisons. Clinical-forensic psychologists practicing in carceral settings focus on providing psychological and risk reduction treatment to detained/incarcerated individuals. They also provide general psychological and forensic mental health evaluation services to detained/incarcerated individuals. Regarding forensic evaluations, violence and recidivism risk assessments to inform risk reduction strategies are perhaps most common. However, in some carceral settings, other types of forensic evaluations may be offered. For example, civil commitment evaluations, adjudicative competence evaluations, and criminal responsibility evaluations are provided in some federal carceral facilities. Further, some carceral facilities—both at the state and federal level—may have a specialization in treating certain mental health conditions, such as substance use disorders, trauma-related disorders, or serious mental illnesses.

There are two factors worthy of additional consideration for clinical-forensic psychologists interested in carceral settings. First is the general bent of a carceral facility versus a true mental health setting. In truth, many carceral settings have made admirable efforts to improve the experience of individuals with mental health challenges behind the walls. Regardless, there exists a perpetual tension between the mission of carceral institutions and providing treatment (Preston et al., 2022). Ultimately, carceral institutions emphasize public safety. Therefore, they prioritize custody, control, and incapacitation (which engenders removal of individuals from their support networks). This focus on public safety often produces conflicting goals with treatment, which emphasizes the autonomy of a patient, works to mitigate power disparities, and works to create supportive environments (Preston et al., 2022). In short, carceral settings may not be ideal for individuals who do not want to think about needing to balance the therapeutic milieu with the need for custody and control.

CARCERAL FACILITIES

States generally have two types of carceral facilities. *Jails* are operated by counties and detain individuals who are awaiting trial on state-level charges, as well as incarcerate offenders serving sentences for less severe crimes. In contrast, *prisons* incarcerate individuals who have been convicted of more serious crimes. Prisons are overseen by a state's Department of Corrections.

At the federal level, *federal detention centers* detain individuals who are awaiting trial on federal charges. *Federal correctional institutions* house individuals who have been convicted of federal crimes. *Federal medical centers* house individuals with specialized medical or mental health needs.

A second consideration is the difficulty level of perpetually working in a carceral setting. Carceral settings pose safety concerns that may not be present in other settings. Further, the nature of clinical work in carceral settings inherently differs from the nature of clinical work in other settings due to the tension mentioned in the paragraph earlier. To this end, psychologists in carceral settings report higher levels of burnout than do individuals in other public service settings (Senter et al., 2010). If you want a low-stress setting where you have some chances to sit back and relax, carceral facilities may not be your optimal setting.

OPPORTUNITIES FOR TEACHING/MENTORSHIP AND RESEARCH

Employment in public sector clinical settings can provide ample opportunities to be involved in teaching and mentorship. Many public sector settings—particularly state hospitals and carceral settings—host psychology practicum students, pre-doctoral interns, and postdoctoral fellows. The same is true of entities that work closely with law enforcement agencies. If you would like the opportunity to mentor students in clinical work or to teach didactic seminars, prioritizing employment at a site that hosts such training programs may be beneficial. To this end, the Student Committee of the American Psychology-Law Society (APA Division 41) regularly updates an index of pre-doctoral internship and postdoctoral fellowship programs on its website that you can review (www.apls-students.org). Many public sector settings also provide opportunities to contribute to research, be it through applying for grants, contributing to program evaluations, or contributing to scholarly publications. For example, numerous influential research articles have been published by forensic psychologists and psychology trainees at California's Patton State Hospital and from the Federal Medical Center at Butner (to name just two esteemed public sector institutions that regularly bolster forensic psychology's research base).

POSITIVES AND NEGATIVES ABOUT PUBLIC SECTOR EMPLOYMENT AS A FORENSIC PSYCHOLOGIST

We would be remiss if we did not provide a balanced take on public sector employment as a clinical-forensic psychologist. Truly, a career in public service can be extremely rewarding (El-Ghoroury, 2009). First, it can be personally rewarding to hold a job that allows you to help others, address social ills, and is consistent with your values. Second, public sector jobs often have attractive benefit packages, such as copious time off, comprehensive medical benefits, solid retirement benefits, potential help with student loan repayment, and eligibility for student loan forgiveness.

However, a career in public service as a clinical-forensic psychologist can also have some downsides. First, a common criticism of public sector settings is that they are underfunded, creating resource shortages and resulting in higher workloads and emotional exhaustion for staff. Research suggests that emotional exhaustion and high workloads are key drivers of burnout among psychologists (McCormack et al., 2018). This has been recently demonstrated regarding clinical-forensic psychologists amid the Competency Services Crisis, with a study showing that half of psychologists working in adjudicative competency contexts felt burned out (with some even considering leaving their jobs) (Ricardo et al., 2025).

A second common criticism of work in public sector settings is that lower yearly compensation might be available versus in private sector settings or blended settings (a mix of public and private sector work). This appears to hold true for clinical-forensic psychologists as well. Though not an exact match in terms of categorization, two recent studies suggest that clinical-forensic psychologists who work only in institutional settings (common in public sector employment) tend to make less on average than do clinical-forensic psychologists who work in private practice settings or who work in blended settings (LaDuke et al., 2024; Neal & Line, 2022). Note, though, that this reduced compensation may be offset somewhat by the potential for loan assistance/forgiveness and attractive benefits packages that can exist in public sector settings (as mentioned earlier).

JOB SEARCH STRATEGIES

So we've convinced you that a clinical-forensic psychology career in public service is the path for you. So how exactly do you go about finding a public service job? Not to worry—we have some tips that may help you in your search. First, as with most job hunting these days, it is helpful to consult job aggregator websites. There are numerous such websites that cater toward public interest jobs; examples are provided in the callout box. Second, city, county, and state governments often host websites where they list open job positions. The federal government also hosts a website with open federal jobs (https://www.usajobs.gov/). Third, it can be helpful to familiarize yourself with the various resources/interventions your desired jurisdiction has along the SIM. This allows you to conduct more targeted monitoring of when certain agencies might have job openings. Fourth (and not to sound cliché), it often is about who you know. Reaching out to your friends and colleagues in public service when you are job hunting—or making sure to maximize your utilization of social media career platforms like LinkedIn—can be fruitful.

JOB AGGREGATOR WEBSITES FOR PUBLIC SERVICE JOBS

- https://www.idealist.org/en
- https://www.careersingovernment.com/
- https://www.publicservicecareers.org/
- https://www.workforgood.org/
- https://www.usajobs.gov/
- https://www.careeronestop.org/
- https://www.linkedin.com/jobs/

CHAPTER TAKEAWAYS

Clinical-forensic psychology careers in public service can be very rewarding. Public servants get to help others and work to mitigate or remedy societal problems, and they can hold jobs that should comport with their values.

With the overlap between mental illness and criminal justice involvement becoming ever more noticeable—and the continued evolution of the field of forensic psychology to address this issue—it is a very exciting time to ponder a career in public service, even with the potential detriments that exist (e.g., burnout, lower pay). If you are interested in a clinical-forensic psychology career in public service, familiarizing yourself with the SIM, exploring job openings in common public sectors settings (public psychiatric hospitals, law enforcement agencies, forensic mental health services, and carceral settings), and following the job search tips we laid out should prove helpful. Now, go forth and serve!

Career Profile: Natalie Anumba, Ph.D., ABPP (Forensic)

Where Are You Currently Working, and What Position Do You Hold?

I work on behalf of a state agency through a contract with a public university, so I wear a few different hats. Because my position is funded through a contract with the Massachusetts Department of Mental Health (DMH), I practice as a forensic psychologist and conduct court-ordered forensic mental health assessments on behalf of DMH at the Worcester Recovery Center and Hospital (a state psychiatric hospital). I am faculty (associate professor) at the University of Massachusetts Chan Medical School, in the Department of Psychiatry, and I serve as Co-director of the Law and Psychiatry Program. All of this is to say that I spend my professional time conducting forensic mental health assessments, providing clinical supervision and training in forensic mental health assessment, and providing administrative support and oversight of the clinical and training activities of the Law and Psychiatry Program.

What Got You Interested in a Career in Working in Public Sector Clinical Practice?

My public sector interest and career trajectory started gradually. I had some exposure to the public sector settings during graduate school, when I did some clinical training in correctional facilities. My pre-doctoral internship further deepened my experience in the correctional setting and provided the opportunity to rotate through a state hospital. My postdoctoral fellowship took place entirely in public sector settings, namely, a state hospital, a correctional hospital, and state courthouse. When I completed my postdoc, I was ready for a career in the public sector and couldn't imagine myself elsewhere. I thus started my career in forensic psychology as a courthouse-based clinician. Public sector service appeals to me because these settings have high needs for mental health services and involve a broad array of clinical presentations; the work is ever-present and always interesting.

What Does an Average Workday Look Like for You, in Terms of Duties and Responsibilities?

It's hard to have "a regular day" as a forensic psychologist! Given the multiple roles I fulfill, there is a great deal of flexibility over how I spend my time, combined with multiple pressing deadlines. My workday consists of some combination of interviewing examinees or collaterals, consulting with treatment providers or legal professionals, reviewing records, writing reports, testifying in court, supervising postdoctoral trainees, developing or leading didactic trainings, academic writing, program administration, and various forms of academic service (committee meetings, reviewing journal manuscripts). There is no way to do all of these in one day, so I tend to dedicate each day out of the workweek to a certain group of tasks (e.g., interviews and consultations on one day, academic and administrative tasks on another). At the beginning of a given day, I will review my calendar for relevant deadlines and meetings, prioritize the necessary tasks, and create a schedule to keep myself on track. Do I stick to the schedule and accomplish everything on the list every day? Absolutely not, I'm human.

What Is the Most Rewarding Aspect of Your Work?

My work is rewarding for its ongoing learning and daily intellectual exercise. In my clinical practice, I enjoy learning about people, discussing things I find intensely interesting (human functioning and behavior), and educating non-clinicians about clinical concepts as applied to specific individuals. In my education and training roles, I have the privilege of working with smart and thoughtful professionals who are diligent, eager to learn, and motivated to improve their practice and the world around them. Finally, in my professional service activities, I have the opportunity to collaborate with colleagues from all over and to participate in projects that move the field forward.

What Have Been Some of the Most Challenging Things to Navigate in Your Work?

One challenging aspect of my work is that forensic mental health practice involves exposure to terrible things, including examinees' histories of trauma and/or wading through the details of appalling allegations. More prosaically, high levels of need for forensic evaluations (and mental health services more generally) means that clinical work makes significant demands on practitioners' time. Academia is also unique in that while there are many ways to engage in teaching, scholarship, and professional service, it is easy to give all of yourself away without realizing it. Therefore, this job requires attention to self-care and active efforts to avoid neglecting life outside of work.

If Someone Wanted to Follow in Your Footsteps, What Advice Would You Give Them?

My first piece of advice is to do some research to find what interests you. As this book demonstrates, "forensic psychologist" is a very broad term that incorporates multiple roles across multiple settings—sometimes even within one job. If you think this field is for you, read and learn about what you find most interesting and appealing, and structure your preparation accordingly. Such research provides an opportunity to begin developing relevant experience early and make yourself a competitive candidate for your chosen career path. What is just as important is that by proceeding in this way, you can identify what you do *not* want to spend your career doing.

Next, and possibly paradoxically, read broadly. Forensic training will necessarily involve immersion in the foundational standards, principles, and texts of the field. However, as I have progressed in my career, I have found enormous benefit from reading and becoming familiar with literature and knowledge developed outside of the specialty (and even outside of the discipline of psychology). Having a broad knowledge base has fueled expertise, critical thinking, creativity, and innovation in my practice.

Finally, be sure to continue your development as a person: take time off to pursue hobbies, explore the world, volunteer, and spend time with your loved ones.

Career Profile: Tallie Armstrong, Ph.D., ABPP (Forensic)

Where Are You Currently Working, and What Position Do You Hold?

Currently, I work with the Commonwealth of Virginia's Department of Behavioral Health and Developmental Services (DBHDS), Office of Forensic Services (OFS). It is a forensic evaluator position; the bulk of my caseload is competency to proceed and sanity evaluations. However, I also complete sexual violence risk and violence risk assessments for our Sexually Violent Predator (SVP) and our not guilty by reason of insanity populations. This position is somewhat distinctive in that it is fully remote, although we occasionally go to jails or facilities to complete court-ordered evaluations. My role is also unique in that I am (and the team of evaluators I work with are) stationed in the administrative branch of our state mental health department, as opposed to being anchored to a specific state hospital. This means we serve any facility that requests our services. My location in the OFS also provides me with a seat at some of the tables where discussions are being had about the trajectory of forensic evaluation and treatment work occurring within our system (e.g., how to manage increasing numbers of evaluations). This position also affords me the opportunity to serve as a peer supervisor to evaluators in the system whose reports were flagged for not meeting the OFS's minimum requirements for report writing. We also consult with facilities and evaluators when particularly challenging cases come along. In addition, I assist with training colleagues by hosting didactics and providing in-service trainings to facilities.

At DBHDS, I also chair the Institutional Review Board (IRB). Since returning to the Virginia system in 2021, I have worked with organizational leadership to create a research infrastructure that can support and promote research. Initially, there was no centralized IRB, and it took a significant amount of extra time and persistence on my part to understand the DBHDS system in order to learn where new ground needed to be traversed versus incorporating existing departments and structure, to find the key players who would need to hear my pitch, and to create an action plan that has ultimately become the groundwork for a solid research infrastructure. Currently, the program is in its infancy, but a typical workload for me involves meeting with organizational leadership to clarify their expectations for what our research infrastructure can provide and my role as the IRB Chair within it; creating policies and procedures; creating easy-to-read documents to support, protect, and promote ethical human-subjects research projects; and reviewing relevant research that comes through our system.

What Got You Interested in a Career in Working in Public Sector Clinical Practice?

I think it's important to point out that many of us do not typically envision a career in public sector work; often, we are thrust into public sector positions very early on in our training because that is where most training opportunities exist. In some ways, I did not inherently have a vision of public sector work when I began walking down the career path of forensic psychologist. Rather, it was through my repeated exposure to and advanced training in this setting (and specifically, strict security state hospitals) that I deepened my interest in advancing my career in this setting. That said, public sector work confers a lot of advantages that maintain my interest! Initially, I enjoyed working in state hospital systems because of the variety of clinical work available. As I began honing my training to be more evaluation-based in nature, I started gravitating toward systems that offered complex cases, which typically meant there was intersectionality between mental illness and violence risk. That intersectionality is what pulled me toward my time at two maximum-security state psychiatric hospitals before I moved into the current position I hold. Another element of public sector work that I have really enjoyed is that despite the rigidity and bureaucratic undertones that are inherent in monolithic, public sector systems, there is a surprising amount of flexibility when you understand the system and find the right people who are interested in new ideas. The cost, of course, is that implementing new ideas takes time and effort that you do not often (or initially, at least) get paid for. In addition, my current public sector job has a lot of benefits attached outside of the actual forensic work itself: full-time remote work, excellent healthcare benefits, access not only to public student loan forgiveness but also state-based loan repayment programs, retirement benefits that include a pension, a high number of paid holidays, and an opportunity to roll over some unused leave time. For positions in Virginia that don't include full-time remote work, most facilities offer evaluators at least one day remote work and/or a compressed schedule. Because of this flexibility, many state-based evaluators in Virginia (myself included) have thriving side private practices.

What Does an Average Workday Look Like for You, in Terms of Duties and Responsibilities?

I think it may be better to couch my answer in what a typical week looks like for me. A typical week usually involves me being assigned three cases for evaluation (sometimes four if I've been assigned a violence risk or sexual violence risk assessment) and then rounding out my time addressing IRB-Chair-related work and all my "other duties as assigned" responsibilities. I often begin the week preparing my cases and sitting in on meetings where I serve as a liaison between a facility's forensic evaluation service and our Office of Forensic Services. By midweek, I have typically completed all my interviews and will spend the remainder of the week writing reports and/or providing feedback to treatment teams, reviewing IRB-protocols and fine-tuning policy and procedure for our research infrastructure, and meeting with my team for our weekly supervision. Other activities that can occur during a typical week include co-facilitating a statewide "office hours," where any evaluator doing state-based work can present and we can discuss various case-related issues, fielding various calls from attorneys or other evaluators, facilitating a didactic or training session, and assisting with peer supervision of colleagues.

What Is the Most Rewarding Aspect of Your Work?

One of the most rewarding aspects of my work is being able to take advantage of the flexibility of the system that I mentioned earlier (in a good way!). If you're motivated and have the time and energy to spare, and if you take the time to learn the system and leaders you're working with, then there's a lot of opportunity available to create some very cool interventions, programs, etc. My pushing to reform the research infrastructure and creating the statewide IRB is the most obvious example of that in my current position. Private sector work certainly has a lot of flexibility, too, but there is something deeply gratifying knowing that I was able to—across multiple state hospitals over the course of my career thus far—navigate those systems and create a program that did not previously exist. In some ways, that gratification ties into a reason I've stayed in the public sector for as long as I have. I have helped create a program that will serve the system and, by extension, the people in Virginia who most need a strong and well-functioning mental health system. I also very much enjoy the variety and complexity of cases that I get to work through because I can work across the entire state, as opposed to one region of the state (as is custom with most state facilities). Public sector psychology work, generally, is also very strongly oriented toward supervision, mentorship, and training, and Virginia's state mental health system is no exception. I have enjoyed receiving quality mentorship, as well as getting to explore mentorship, supervision, and training not just in a traditional sense (i.e., with postdoctoral fellowship supervision) but also as a peer mentor and in supervising individuals across DBHDS who are interested in research.

What Have Been Some of the Most Challenging Things to Navigate in Your Work?

Even though most of us are steeped in public sector work as a byproduct of our training, it certainly does not have to be a path that all of us take. Public sector work can be thankless and grueling, and sometimes it pays very poorly. As I mentioned earlier, state mental health systems contain an inherent degree of rigidity, and therefore, change of any meaningful sort rarely occurs quickly. Maintaining the patience and motivation to push one's agenda or ideas forward in that kind of an environment requires a lot of stamina and a lot of unrecognized hours of work. In addition, many state mental health systems are under an extraordinary amount of strain due to the "competency crisis" (among other issues) that has resulted in a shortage of evaluators compared to evaluations needed. Because DBHDS's budget is controlled by Virginia's General Assembly, and DBHDS is so large, it can be very challenging for OFS to effectively compete for resources with other areas of the organization who have similar needs (e.g., the substance abuse branch of DBHDS working to manage opioid addiction). As a result, many evaluators are asked to take on more cases than they would normally, resulting in burnout. As a professional who has seen others work through burnout and who has experienced it myself, it can be a challenge to see the value of your professional worth when you're in a system that may not fully appreciate the "gatekeeping" function you serve as an evaluator or treatment provider. Also, even though I have had an extraordinary amount of success in creating research infrastructure in my current position, it has been an eye-opening experience that not all individuals in leadership positions understand the merits of having human subjects research protections and the benefits that can be gleaned from supporting a functional research infrastructure.

If Someone Wanted to Follow in Your Footsteps, What Advice Would You Give Them?

The first thing I would say is never take public sector work at face value. I mean that in a good way! That is, look beyond the monolithic and rigid nature of the system. Find the people and the part of the system that is open to flexibility. For example, if you don't like a particular job or position, figure out how to work with the system to grow a position that you want. In my current role, I see how there is a strong need in our system to improve our NGRI-conditional release process. Thus, I am currently working with our office to see how we can make some important changes. I would also recommend truly learning the system in which you operate. That can be challenging, especially if you're housed out of one facility that is part of a larger structure. However, psychology public sector employees are always looking for young individuals who want to learn the system so they can start to figure out how to improve it. Finally, I encourage you to do some self-reflection and determine whether working in that kind of a system will truly meet your professional needs. Public sector work can certainly provide a lot of upward mobility, but that mobility can occur in fits and starts and, as I said earlier, can occur very slowly. If maintaining patience and stamina in a system that can be very unkind to evaluators and providers in terms of workload is difficult, it is okay to decide public sector work may not be a long-term fit for you.

REFERENCES

Abreu, D., Parker, T. W., Noether, C. D., Steadman, H. J., & Case, B. (2017). Revising the paradigm for jail diversion for people with mental illness and substance use disorders: Intercept 0. *Behavioral Sciences & Law*, *35*(5–6), 380–395. https://doi.org/10.1002/bsl.2300

Addington v. Texas, 441 U.S. 418. (1979).

American Psychological Association. (2022, May). *Police and public safety psychology*. https://www.apa.org/ed/graduate/specialize/police

Bonfine, N., & Nadler, N. (2019). The perceived impact of sequential intercept mapping on communities collaborating to address adults with mental illness in the criminal justice system. *Administration and Policy in Mental Health*, *46*(5), 569–579. https://doi.org/10.1007/s10488-019-00936-z

Bratina, M. P. (Ed.). (2023). *Forensic mental health: Framing integrated solutions*. Routledge. https://doi.org/10.4324/9781003120186

Cooper, A. (2013). The ongoing correctional chaos in criminalizing mental illness: The realignments effects on California jails. *Hastings Women's Law Journal*, *24*(2), 339–362.

Corey, D. M., & Zelig, M. (2020). *Evaluations of police suitability and fitness for duty*. Oxford University Press.

Crisanti, A. S., Fairfax-Columbo, J., Duran, D., Rosenbaum, N. A., Melendrez, B., Trujillo, I., Earheart, J. A., & Tinney, M. (2022). Evaluation of ongoing Crisis Intervention Team (CIT) training for law enforcement using the ECHO model. *Journal of Police and Criminal Psychology*, *37*(4), 863–875. https://doi.org/10.1007/s11896-022-09529-3

El-Ghoroury, N. H. (2009). The benefits of a public service career. *gradPSYCH Magazine*, *7*(4). https://www.apa.org/gradpsych/2009/11/matters

Gowensmith, W. N. (2019). Resolution or resignation: The role of forensic mental health professionals amidst the competency services crisis. *Psychology, Public Policy, and Law*, *25*(1), 1–14. https://psycnet.apa.org/doi/10.1037/law0000190

Gowensmith, W. N., Frost, L. E., Speelman, D.W., & Therson, D. E. (2016). Lookin' for beds in all the wrong places: Outpatient competency restoration as a promising approach to modern challenges. *Psychology, Public Policy, and Law*, *22*(3), 293–305. https://psycnet.apa.org/doi/10.1037/law0000088

Griffin, P. A., Heilbrun, K., Mulvey, E. P., DeMatteo, D., & Schubert, C. A. (Eds.). (2015). *The Sequential Intercept Model and criminal justice: Promoting community alternatives for individuals with serious mental illness*. Oxford University Press.

Heilbrun, K., & DeMatteo, D. (Eds.). (in press). *Community-based psychological services for justice-involved individuals*. Oxford University Press.

Kois, L. E., Murrie, D. C., Gowensmith, W. N., & Packer, I. K. (2023). A public health perspective to reform the competence to stand trial system. *Psychiatric Services*, *74*(12), 1289–1290. https://doi.org/10.1176/appi.ps.20230079

Kois, L. E., Potts, H., Cox, J., & Zapf, P. (2024). Court-reported competence to proceed data across the United States. *Law and Human Behavior*, *48*(3), 182–202. https://doi.org/10.1037/lhb0000565

Kuehn, B. M. (2014). Criminal justice becomes front line for mental health care. *Journal of the American Medical Association*, *311*(19), 1953–1954. https://doi.org/10.1001/jama.2014.4578

LaDuke, C., DeMatteo, D., Brank, E. M., & Kavanaugh, A. (2024). Training, practice, and career considerations in forensic psychology: Results from a field survey of clinical and non-clinical professionals in the United States. *Frontiers in Psychology*, *15*, 1439874. https://doi.org/10.3389/fpsyg.2024.1439874

Lamb, H. R., & Weinberger, L. E. (2020). Deinstitutionalization and other factors in the criminalization of persons with serious mental illness and how it is being addressed. *CNS Spectrums*, *25*(2), 173–180. https://doi.org/10.1017/s1092852919001524

Lee, C. (2024, March 20). Public safety psychologists: Understanding their role and how they can support your department. *American Police Beat*. https://apbweb.com/2024/03/public-safety-psychologists/

Luxton, D. D., & Niemi, J. (2020). Implementation and evaluations of videoconferencing for forensic competency evaluation. *Telemedicine and e-Health*, *26*(7), 929–934. https://doi.org/10.1089/tmj.2019.0150

Manguno-Mire, G. M., Thompson, J. W., Jr., Shore, J. H., Croy, C. D., Artecona, J. F., & Pickering, J. W. (2007). The use of telemedicine to evaluate competency to stand trial: A preliminary randomized controlled study. *The Journal of the American Academy of Psychiatry and the Law*, *35*(4), 481–489.

McCormack, H. M., MacIntyre, T. E., O'Shea, D., Herring, M. P., & Campbell, M. J. (2018). The prevalence and cause(s) of burnout among applied psychologists: A systematic review. *Frontiers in Psychology*, *9*, 1897. https://doi.org/10.3389/fpsyg.2018.01897

Melton, G. B., Petrila, J., Poythress, N. G., Slobogin, C., Otto, R. K., Mossman, D., & Condie, L. O. (2018). *Psychological evaluations for the courts: A handbook for mental health professionals and lawyers* (4th ed.). The Guilford Press.

Monfared, J. (2022, February 10). What is police psychology and is it a career for you? *CONCEPT The Business of Practice Blog*. https://concept.paloaltou.edu/resources/business-of-practice-blog/what-is-police-psychology-and-is-it-a-career-for-you

Mumford, E. A., Liu, W., & O'Leary. (2024). U.S. law enforcement officers' stress, job satisfaction, job performance, and resilience: A national sample. *Police Quarterly*, *28*(1), 104–126. https://doi.org/10.1177/10986111241253851

Munetz, M., & Griffin, P. A. (2006). Use of the Sequential Intercept Model as an approach to decriminalization of people with serious mental illness. *Psychiatric Services*, *57*(4), 544–549. https://doi.org/10.1176/ps.2006.57.4.544

Murrie, D. C., Gowensmith, W. N., Kois, L. E., & Packer, I. K. (2023). Evaluations of competence to stand trial are evolving amid a national "competency crisis." *Behavioral Sciences & the Law*, *41*(5), 310–325. https://doi.org/10.1002/bsl.2620

Neal, T. M. S., & Line, E. N. (2022). Income, demographics, and life experiences of clinical-forensic psychologists in the United States. *Frontiers in Psychology*, *13*, 910672. https://doi.org/10.3389/fpsyg.2022.910672

O'Connor v. Donaldson, 422 U.S. 563 (1975).

Osborn, L. A. (2009). From beauty to despair: The rise and fall of the American state mental hospital. *Psychiatric Quarterly*, *80*(4), 219–231. https://doi.org/10.1007/s11126-009-9109-3

Panza, N., Kelly, J., & Walsh, W. (2024). Annual wellness visits for police and public safety officers: Current practices among mental health professionals and considerations for future program development. *Journal of Police and Criminal Psychology*. https://doi.org/10.1007/s11896-024-09724-4

Pinals, D. A., & Callahan, L. (2020). Evaluation and restoration of competence to stand trial: Intercepting the forensic system using the Sequential Intercept Model. *Psychiatric Services*, *71*(7), 698–705. https://doi.org/10.1176/appi.ps.201900484

Preston, A. G., Rosenberg, A., Schlesinger, P., & Blankenship, K. M. (2022). "I was reaching out for help and they did not help me": Mental healthcare in the carceral state." *Health and Justice*, *10*, 23. https://doi.org/10.1186/s40352-022-00183-9

Reingle Gonzalez, J. M., & Connell, N. M. (2014). Mental health of prisoners: Identifying barriers to mental health treatment and medication continuity. *American Journal of Public Health*, *104*(12), 2328–2333. https://doi.org/10.2105/AJPH.2014.302043

Ricardo, M. M., Formon, D. L., Bailey, C. A., & Boccaccini, M. T. (2025). The competency crisis and forensic evaluator burnout. *Psychological Services*. Online publication. https://doi.org/10.1037/ser0000965

Rotter, M., & Compton, M. (2022). Criminal legal involvement: A cause and consequence of social determinants of health. *Psychiatric Services*, *73*(1), 108–111. https://doi.org/10.1176/appi.ps.202000741

Rushing, E., Ao, B., Dean, M. M., & Purcell, D. (2020, October 27). Walter Wallace Jr., 27, a 'family man' with many mental health crisis and encounters with police. *The Philadelphia Inquirer*. https://www.inquirer.com/news/walter-wallace-jr-philadelphia-mental-health-20201027.html?srsltid=AfmBOorqjLbLDoYrnlMAXdtM7umdj8_K7G9vOnZzbUyIYZxQ0Ba_2GSw

Scott, C. K., Dennis, M. L., Grella, C. E., Mischel, A. F., & Carnevale, J. (2021). The impact of the opioid crisis on U.S. state prison systems. *Health & Justice*, *9*, 17. https://doi.org/10.1186/s40352-021-00143-9

Segal, A. G., Frasco, R., & Sisti, D. A. (2018). County jail or psychiatric hospital? Ethical challenges in correctional mental health care. *Qualitative Health Research*, *28*(6), 963–976. https://doi.org/10.1177/1049732318762370

Senter, A., Morgan, R. D., Serna-McDonald, C., & Bewley, M. (2010). Correctional psychologist burnout, job satisfaction, and life satisfaction. *Psychological Services*, *7*(3), 190–201. https://psycnet.apa.org/doi/10.1037/a0020433

Swanson, L., Nelson, V., Comartin, E. B., Kubiak, S., Putans, L., Hambrick, N., Ray, B., Tillander, L., Washington, A., Butkiewicz, R., & Costello, M. (2023). Assessing county-level behavioral health and justice systems with the Sequential Intercept

Model practices, leadership, and expertise scorecard. *Community Mental Health Journal*, *59*(3), 578–594. https://doi.org/10.1007/s10597-022-01042-5

Wik, A., Hollen, V., & Fisher, W. H. (2020). Forensic patients in state psychiatric hospitals: 1999–2016. *CNS Spectrums*, *25*(2), 196–206. https://doi.org/10.1017/S1092852919001044

Yeo, Y., Johnson, R., & Heng, C. (2022). The public health approach to the worsening opioid crisis in the United States call for harm reduction strategies to mitigate the harm from opioid addiction and overdose deaths. *Military Medicine*, *187*(9–10), 244–247. https://doi.org/10.1007/s10597-022-01042-5

CHAPTER 7

The Private Life

An Overview of Individual and Group Private Practices

Do you want agency in your day-to-day work life? Do you want to be able to prioritize your own career vision instead of having to prioritize an employer's? Do you like the idea of having a flexible work schedule and not having to punch the clock and keep the same 9-to-5(ish) work schedule every day? Do you value being able to be selective about the forensic mental health assessment referrals that you take on? How about being able to pursue your varied interests and take advantage of myriad professional opportunities without worrying about whether you need your boss' approval to do so? Want the ability to better manage your caseload and not be subject to feeling overworked, overburdened, overlooked, and burned out? Do you strive to attain the seemingly elusive "work-life" balance concept everyone talks about? If you answered "yes" to any of—or all—of these questions, private practice might be the career setting for you! This chapter will predominantly discuss what it is like to "be your own boss" in clinical-forensic psychology. It will provide an overview of private forensic psychology practice, including its advantages and drawbacks. We will also briefly review options for individuals who are interested in testing the private practice waters but who may not be ready to fully commit to it.

I WANT TO BE MY OWN BOSS: AN OVERVIEW OF PRIVATE PRACTICE

Private practice in clinical-forensic psychology often differs distinctly from more traditional private psychotherapy or psychological assessment practices. First, the majority of clinical-forensic psychology private practice occurs

DOI: 10.4324/9781003408857-10

outside the purview of health insurance/managed care. Instead of billing an insurance company, which involves copious paperwork to justify reimbursement for services, forensic psychologists generally invoice the referral source for the services they provided (typically, attorneys or courts) (Mart, 2006). As you might imagine, this substantially cuts down on the administrative burden of running a private clinical psychology practice. It also typically means that forensic psychologists are receiving higher payment for their services since the prices are not set by insurance companies.

Second, private practice clinical-forensic psychologists typically have a practice that is heavy on forensic mental health assessment. Unlike a therapy-focused practice, clinical-forensic psychologists do not typically maintain consistent, long-term relationships with the individuals they serve. Unlike a therapeutic assessment-focused practice, clinical-forensic psychologists who conduct forensic mental health assessments are not focused on informing treatment plans. Instead, clinical-forensic psychologists conduct evaluations to inform psycholegal questions. Further, the client in a forensic mental health assessment is not the evaluee but rather the referral source (typically, an attorney, a court, or an administrative agency) (Heilbrun, 2001).

PRACTICE NOTE

Even if most of a clinical-forensic psychologist's private practice concerns forensic mental health assessment—or psychological assessments for the courts—clinical-forensic psychologists are often called upon to do more "traditional" assessment and treatment. Common populations that clinical-forensic psychologists may work with in a therapeutic role include sex offenders, domestic violence offenders, individuals with substance abuse and legal involvement, and children and families with legal involvement (Mart, 2006).

Third, the common end results of forensic mental health assessments vary. They may result in a simple phone call or videoconference where you provide an attorney valuable information, but ultimately, they do not ask you to move forward with drafting anything. They may result in you drafting a letter for an attorney's file, perhaps a more formalized version of the former. Alternatively, they may result in a written report, but you are never called upon to testify. Alternatively again, they may result in a written report and testimony in a deposition, hearing, or trial. Regardless, forensic psychologists conducting forensic mental health assessments do not complete running therapy notes. If a report is requested, it serves as the primary form of documentation and memorialization of the services rendered (Otto et al., 2014). If no report is requested (or required), the only documentation/memorialization of the services rendered lies in communications between the attorney

and the clinical-forensic psychologist or in draft materials prepared in antici-
pation of litigation; such documentation is generally privileged and not dis-
coverable under Federal Rule of Civil Procedure 26(b) (2024) or corollary
state rules of civil procedure.

Fourth, many forensic mental health assessments may not take place in a
traditional office setting but instead in institutional settings or at an attorney's office. Depending on the type of cases a clinical-forensic psychologist
elects to take, this may diminish the need to rent and maintain an independent office.

PRACTICE NOTE

Clinical-forensic psychologists with primary forensic mental health assessment practices may not need to invest in and rely on expensive practice management software.
They also may not need to maintain a private office. This can significantly reduce
overhead cost as compared to other clinical psychologists.

ADVANTAGES OF FORENSIC PSYCHOLOGY PRIVATE PRACTICE

Greater Professional Flexibility

Perhaps the chief benefit of being in private practice in clinical-forensic
psychology is that the "world is your oyster." Unlike being an employee
of a company, agency, or institution—where psychologists generally receive
defined job descriptions—the limits of job duties in private practice are
solely imposed by the practitioner. Many private practitioners have their
hands in multiple pots. For example, they may conduct forensic mental
health assessments Monday to Thursday, partner with a university-based colleague on research and publications on Tuesday evenings, teach a class on
forensic psychology at a local college or university as an adjunct professor
on Wednesday evenings, and provide counseling in a correctional institution
on Fridays (DeMatteo et al., 2020).

Similarly, being an employee of a company, agency, or institution often
results in working in a defined role. For example, the sole job duties of a
clinical-forensic psychologist employed at a state forensic hospital might be
to conduct civil commitment, adjudicative competence, and mental state at
the time of the offense evaluations. This places them in the sole role of evaluative expert. These experts are objective and are neutral, meaning they should
be uninterested in the outcome of a case and are not aligned with any side.

Further, private practitioners may have greater flexibility in the expert roles they adopt. For example, a private practitioner may be approached by an attorney solely to review records and provide some guidance as to how best to proceed in a case. A private practitioner may also be approached to review the work of another expert to identify potential shortfalls or flaws (if any) in that expert's work and to assist the retaining attorney in drafting cross-examination questions. Additionally, a forensic psychologist may be called upon to assist an attorney in navigating jury selection. In these scenarios, the forensic psychologist acts as a consulting expert. They maintain objectivity, but they are allied with a particular side and work specifically to help and guide them.

As a third role, a private practitioner may have a particular area of research expertise that makes them well-versed to educate judges and juries on a particular topic, such as the limitations of human memory or factors that contribute to false confessions. In this instance, the forensic psychologist would be acting as a teaching expert. Finally, forensic psychologists may be approached to provide testimony to lawmakers on key forensic mental health issues, such as the impact of sex offender notification and registration laws on offender reentry and public safety (Thompson & Frumkin, 2023). Here, the forensic psychologist serves as a teaching expert in the realm of public policy.

As a note, none of the aforementioned is to suggest that forensic psychologists who work outside of private practice settings cannot serve in multiple expert roles. Rather, it only suggests that typical "employee" status creates some restrictions on how a forensic psychologist can practice.

In private practice, forensic psychologists can choose not only the *type* of work they would like to engage in but also *when* and *where* they would like to work. They are not beholden to specified hours or to specified settings. Busy during the week but need to schedule an evaluation? A private practitioner may be able to schedule a weekend evaluation session. Big fan of Brazilian Jiu Jitsu but prefer a daytime class as nighttime classes are too crowded? Hate going to the grocery store during peak times? A private practitioner can work on a report in the morning from their local coffee shop (while being sure to protect confidentiality), head to the gym for a noon Brazilian Jiu Jitsu class, grocery shop on their way home, and resume working on the report in the evening.

Greater Selectivity in the Referrals They Accept

A second key benefit of being a private practitioner is greater *selectivity* in the types of referrals taken. Forensic psychologists who are "employees" typically have cases assigned to them by a supervisor. They may have very limited ability to turn down cases they do not want to take. They may also have limited ability to ask to take on cases that involve new and interesting referral questions. In contrast, private practitioners can dictate the breadth—or the narrowness—of the referral questions they accept. Instead of being constrained to only a few questions, some private practice forensic psychologists may have an expansive practice. For example, they may take myriad criminal-forensic referral questions with both juveniles and adults, such as adjudicative competence, competence to waive *Miranda* Rights, mental state at the time of the offense, recidivism risk assessment, and mitigation. They may also take referrals that are more administrative in nature, such as fitness for duty evaluations or disability determinations. Further, they may take civil-forensic referral questions, such as determination of psychological injury in tort cases.

Greater Freedom in How They Structure and Carry Out Forensic Evaluations

As a final note on flexibility, private practitioners are better able to dictate how they conduct forensic evaluations. For example, research suggests that across surveys, forensic psychologists endorse using a variety of testing measures in their evaluative practice (see Archer et al., 2016). Further, there are many tests that measure similar constructs that appear to meet admissibility criteria in United States courts (see Neal et al., 2019). Despite this, being an employee of a company, agency, or organization may come with constraints as to what measures can be used. For example, a particular employer may provide access to specific measures of personality, violence risk assessment, and symptom validity; these may not be the measures that, left to their own choices, a particular forensic psychologist would favor. Being self-employed allows for greater discretion in what measures to use, so long as the measures meet ethical standards for psychologists and admissibility standards for courts. However, note that purchasing testing measures, scoring software, and other testing materials is an overhead cost of running a business, meaning this cost is on the private practitioner as a proprietor. This is not the case when a clinical-forensic psychologist is an employee.

Pay

Though increased freedom and discretion are key motivating factors for forensic psychologists entering private practice, an increase in earning potential is another extremely salient factor. Given increased costs of living, debt crises, and other financial strains people face daily, compensation is often a critical consideration in choosing a career path. To this end, private practitioners have the potential to make more money than their peers who are employees. For example, research from Neal and Line (2022) and LaDuke et al. (2024) suggests private practice forensic psychologists make significantly more money than their counterparts who work in institutional or university settings.

CHALLENGES OF FORENSIC PSYCHOLOGY PRIVATE PRACTICE

As indicated earlier, private practice in forensic psychology has many advantages. However, as with anything, there are simultaneous downsides. Some of these downsides are typical of any type of clinical psychology private practice, including administrative duties and needing to develop business management skills. For example, in reflecting on her entry into private practice, clinical psychologist Deborah Vineberg noted that in addition to the hat of "clinical psychologist," she also had to wear the hats of "accountant, public relations person, cleaning lady, insurance policy expert, receptionist, real estate agent, financial analyst, bill collector, and office manager" (2005, p. 90). Another generalized challenge of clinical psychology private practice includes needing to be more proactive in personal financial planning. Full-time private practitioners are typically responsible for securing their own health insurance—which can be expensive—and do not have access to employer-sponsored retirement programs. However, other challenges are more specific to the practice of forensic psychology, detailed later.

Having to Obtain Referrals and Market Oneself

As exciting as being your own boss can be, it also means that you are solely responsible for generating the business that sustains you (Thompson & Frumkin, 2023). This can seem like a formidable task, particularly for early-career forensic psychologists or for forensic psychologists who are new to a jurisdiction (DeMatteo et al., 2020). However, there are multiple business development and marketing strategies in forensic psychology that are effective in building a referral base. Key marketing activities might include doing things to encourage word-of-mouth marketing (e.g., such as doing high-quality work, enhancing visibility through publishing); establishing a website; and sending cover letters to lawyers, law agencies (e.g., such as a local Public Defender's Office), and law firms (Melton et al., 2018). Further, giving talks to local bar associations or legal groups can increase visibility

(Mart, 2006). Additionally, private practitioners often benefit from tracking their referrals, and they should be flexible in pursuing new referral strategies if their existing strategies are not yielding sufficient results (Mart, 2007).

Being on an Island

As may be obvious at this point in the book, forensic mental health assessments can be nuanced and complex. The ability to readily consult with peers is extremely beneficial. Psychologists who work in settings where multiple forensic psychologists are on staff—such as in a state forensic hospital or in a court clinic—have coworkers with whom they can easily consult. Unfortunately, private practitioners may not have easy access to professional consultation (Thompson & Frumkin, 2023).

This does not mean that consultation is *not available* to private practitioners; it simply means that they may have to actively seek out this support. To this end, forensic psychologists in private practice might make it a point to build their professional networks. Thankfully, there are many ways to do so, including joining professional organizations and attending their conferences (e.g., American Psychology-Law Society or International Association of Forensic Mental Services), joining forensic psychology listservs, attending continuing education seminars, or pursuing board certification via the American Board of Forensic Psychology.

Difficulty Maintaining Work-Life Balance (The Profit Incentive)

On the opposite side of the coin, private practitioners sometimes face the problem of having *too much demand* for their services. Because referral sources may come and go, private practitioners may feel pressure to take all referrals that present themselves to maintain steady profit. After all, who knows when the stream of referrals may suddenly run dry?

The pressure to entertain all cases that come your way presents two key challenges. First, it is incumbent on forensic psychologists to practice within the realm of their competence. Private practice might compel some forensic psychologists to be more "flexible" with the cases they take than they truly should be. In other words, private practice forensic psychologists may feel tension to take a referral that stretches or exceeds the bounds of their competence (Thompson & Frumkin, 2023). Second, being too encompassing of referrals that come your way can lead to burnout. The work of a forensic psychologist is intellectually stimulating, which is a plus! However, it is also cognitively and, at times, emotionally, taxing. When a forensic psychologist is an employee, there is typically an upper limit—imposed by an employer—on how much they can be expected to work. When a forensic psychologist is self-employed, though, it is on them to establish the upper limit.

Pressure for Repeat Business

Private practitioners may face pressure to secure repeat business. This can generate tension for forensic psychologists who are supposed to reach objective opinions. For court-ordered evaluations where a forensic psychologist was not retained by an adversarial party, remaining objective may be easier. For party-retained evaluations, however, a psychologist may be motivated—likely subconsciously—to obtain findings and reach opinions that are advantageous to the party that retained them. This is termed *adversarial allegiance,* and it has been well-documented in the research literature (for a review, see Murrie & Boccaccini, 2015). Further, adversarial allegiance can lead to a psychologist obtaining a reputation as a "hired gun," which can raise serious questions about a forensic psychologist's objectivity and integrity and substantially undermine their professional credibility (Mart, 2006). Therefore, it is imperative that private practitioners educate themselves on common biases in forensic mental health assessment and take steps to mitigate those biases (see, e.g., Guarnera et al., 2017; Neal et al., 2022; Zapf & Dror, 2017).

Knowing Your Worth

A final challenge of private practice in forensic psychology is knowing one's worth—i.e., setting rates. Unlike being an employee whose salary, hourly rate, and promotion or bonus structure is determined by their employer, private practitioners are often able to choose their own rates. (Note that there are some exceptions where an organization sets a rate that a forensic psychologist must agree to if they want to secure the referral source). When private practitioners are able to set their own rates, it can be daunting! Will you set your rate too high and deter referrals? Will you set your rate too low and undervalue yourself? Should you offer to do an evaluation for a flat fee, or is an hourly fee appropriate? Should you cap the amount you charge for the evaluation? Should a retainer be required? What about cancellation or no-show fees? Should you do any *pro bono* or "low bono" work (i.e., work in which you make a conscious decision to charge less than your normal rate to make your services accessible)? There is little guidance in the field around setting rates and billing practices (Melton et al., 2018). However, doing market research to determine what other forensic psychologists in the area might charge, consulting with your professional network, and adjusting your rates as you obtain new information are all valuable tools for navigating rate setting.

A TASTE OF THE PRIVATE LIFE: GROUP PRACTICES AND PART-TIME PRIVATE PRACTICE

If the earlier discussion made you shudder, you are not alone! Starting your own business can be quite overwhelming. Not all forensic psychologists feel comfortable heading out on their own without first getting their sea legs under them. Thankfully, there are two settings in which you can get a glimpse of what it might be like to work in private practice—*group practice* and *part-time private practice*.

Group Practices

Group practices allow for multiple psychologists or healthcare professionals to share both resources and the burdens of running a business. Though group practice structures, philosophies, and makeup can vary widely, they share the common theme of a team of individuals supporting each other instead of a practitioner being solely responsible for supporting the services they provide (Habben, 2005). Group practices provide forensic psychologists with opportunities for consistent support, guidance, mentorship, and supervision. This may be particularly helpful for forensic psychologists who specialized later in their training or those who may not have as much in-the-field experience as they would like (Mart, 2006).

Group practices also offer readily accessible consultation with adept peers, particularly group practices that have multiple specialty areas (Thompson & Frumkin, 2023). For example, an individual in a group practice who specializes in assessing adjudicative competency may encounter a challenging case where both a psychotic disorder and neurodevelopmental issues are in play. Rather than pass on the case, the psychologist may opt to take the case and seek consultation from a neuropsychologist who is also in the practice. Further, peers in a group practice can help prep each other for testimony or consult on ethical dilemmas (Thompson & Frumkin, 2023).

Part-Time Private Practice

For all the excitement that "being your own boss" can bring, establishing a full-time private practice in forensic psychology can be unnerving. Further, it may seem a particularly gargantuan task for early-career forensic psychologists, who often struggle with the notion that they are now "experts" who are independently responsible for their work product (see, e.g., Cox et al., 2017). As some might say, "The struggle is real."

For those who are considering private practice but are apprehensive about going all in, testing the waters by establishing a part-time private practice may present a good solution, particularly because it takes time to build a solid referral base that can sustain a full-time private practice (Clay, 2009). As such, building a practice while collecting a steady paycheck from an employer can prove much less challenging.

Part-time private practice requires some level of professional flexibility—and an employer who does not restrict you from maintaining a side practice. Some psychologists establish their forensic practice in the evenings or on weekends. Other psychologists can work a compressed schedule at their primary job to free up a weekday for their part-time practice. Still others have a job that allows more inherent flexibility (e.g., academia). Part-time practice may be particularly attractive for individuals who would enjoy additional side income but who do not want to invest in the level of infrastructure that full-time forensic psychologists might (e.g., office space, expansive testing materials). As the main source of income is not private practice, part-time private practice forensic psychologists can be more selective in the cases they take. For example, a part-time private practitioner may choose only to take cases where the evaluation can be conducted in an institutional setting or to avoid cases that require comprehensive testing given the cost of testing materials and scoring software.

Part-time private practice may also be particularly attractive for individuals who are interested in taking on a limited set of referral questions and/or referral questions that are uncommon. For example, an individual who specializes in evaluations of capacity to waive *Miranda* Rights may hold a full-time job and only take referrals for this specific referral question. Capacity to waive *Miranda* Rights evaluations are sought much less frequently than other types of evaluations, such as adjudicative competency. As such, the pressure to complete many evaluations—which is unlikely given the referral context—is low.

CHAPTER SUMMARY

Private practice in forensic psychology is distinct from therapeutically oriented private practice and tends to be heavy on forensic mental health assessment, although a variety of professional activities can be pursued. The decision to move into full-time private practice can feel imposing! Chief advantages that private practice in forensic psychology provide include greater professional and personal freedom and greater earning potential. However, potential challenges of private practice in forensic psychology include increased potential for professional isolation, sole responsibility for building a referral base and a sustainable business, pressure to obtain repeat business or to overwork oneself, and rate setting. For those forensic psychologists who are not yet invested in moving into full-time private practice but who would like to test the waters, joining a group private practice or pursuing a part-time private practice may be good options.

Career Profile: Heath Hodges, Ph.D., M.L.S., ABPP (Forensic)

Where Are You Currently Working, and What Position Do You Hold?

I currently work in two positions: one as a private practitioner for my own business (Best Forensic Practice, LLC in the Richmond, Virginia area) and one as a forensic evaluator for a non-profit organization (Netcare Access in Columbus, Ohio). For my private work, I primarily conduct forensic mental health evaluations in administrative (e.g., fitness for duty), civil (e.g., personal injury), and criminal (e.g., insanity, competence to stand trial) settings. I also provide consultation services to attorneys looking to contend with unfavorable mental health evaluations. For Netcare, I mostly conduct remote competency to stand trial evaluations.

What Got You Interested in a Career in Working in Private-Sector Clinical Practice?

I had always been curious about the private sector. It seemed like a fantasy job without any clear path to success. For this reason, it intimidated me. My decision to seriously pursue private practice was initially inspired by negative experiences in the public sector. I experienced many frustrations in this setting. I was disheartened by employers' focus on profit over quality care, distasteful politics, disproportionate work-to-pay, and lack of accountability. These frustrations led to dissatisfaction, burnout, and eventually, resentment. These feelings gave way to curiosity and self-education about something that might be better. The more I learned about private practice, the keener my interest and sharper my ambition for this type of work became.

What Does an Average Workday Look Like for You, in Terms of Duties and Responsibilities?

I try to bookend my workdays with an hour of leisure on each end. For mornings, this might be enjoying two cups of coffee, reading *The New York Times*, or "doom scrolling." It involves an early morning workout fewer times than I prefer. My brain gets plenty hot, but it takes a minute to warm up. My first work hour is dedicated to tasks that have a lighter cognitive load, like checking emails, populating invoices, or other administrative tasks. I reserve more taxing duties for the mid-band of the day. This is when I conduct interviews, write reports, and schedule meetings with attorneys. I try to end the day with relatively easier tasks, like scoring tests, reviewing records, scheduling future appointments, and sorting out lingering emails from the day. It is necessary for me to decompress and readjust to nonwork. Apart from preference, this is key to me getting to sleep. I do my best to avoid "working to bed" by incorporating an hour to wind down. This is my favorite time to indulge in some leisure reading (or audiobooks) or television viewing. It involves a late-day workout fewer times than I prefer.

What Is the Most Rewarding Aspect of Your Work?

The rewards include negative absences and positive additions. I am spared the annoyances (or perhaps horrors) of the public sector, from organizational shackling to interpersonal dramas. In place of this, I gain autonomy, power, and unhindered opportunity. I have noticed that my professional success is directly and positively correlated to my enjoyment of the work. And I enjoy this work the most when I can adhere to my own ideas of ethics, innovation, and progress. The so-called "tricks of the trade" in private practice are coveted by many but shared by few who have such specialized knowledge. I was lucky enough to enjoy mentorship as I climbed into the private sector, and I find it rewarding to do the same for aspiring private practitioners.

What Have Been Some of the Most Challenging Things to Navigate in Your Work?

Initially, the most challenging aspect of private practice was figuring it all out. The learning curve is steep and high but worth it. It is continually challenging to stay abreast of evolving standards of practice, particularly the business side of it. Without the oversight of critical departments in the public sector, like Human Resources or Legal Affairs, it is my responsibility to know if I am complying with tax filing requirements, licensing renewal deadlines, and modified legal requirements. It is challenging to navigate potentially unethical conduct by other forensic practitioners. Often the situation is ambiguous, the severity is subjective, or the appropriate response is unclear. Just as puzzling can be the answer to questions about business ethics, such as appropriate contracting and billing practices. Self-motivation is imperative to success, and it is not always easy to sustain. It is a constant necessity to maintain a healthy measure of self-care, which can intermittently be quite challenging.

If Someone Wanted to Follow in Your Footsteps, What Advice Would You Give Them?

Before diving into private practice, be sure to do your research. Consult with other practitioners, read books on business management (not just psychology books on private practice), generate a detailed and realistic business plan, estimate start-up expenses, and retain an excellent tax professional. Remember and accept that any plunge into business, no matter how thoughtful the plan, will involve a degree of risk. The best anyone can do is to make the risk a calculated one. To keep the business thriving, it is paramount to do good work. In my opinion, this is the best strategy for advertising one's services. A client who values your work will call again, and they will tell all their friends to call you when they have similar needs. I find it just as valuable to split my time among a variety of tasks and evaluation types. This keeps me fresh, interested, and motivated. It is important to stay professionally involved and connected. Consume (and produce) research. Attend presentations and workshops. Conduct professional trainings. Involve yourself with professional organizations, like Division 41 (Psychology and Law) of the American Psychological Association or the American Board of Forensic Psychology. Continue to consult with other colleagues, whose ethics, practices, and personalities you respect. Remember your principles and stick to what you value. I value good work, a reasonable workload, work-life balance, my physical health, and my well-being. There is no employer or supervisor to hold me to those goals, and in private practice, it can be easy to forget or neglect our principles. Listen to your gut, perform self-assessments (e.g., "Am I working too much? Am I sleeping enough?"), and modify your behavior accordingly. This will avoid burnout and, most importantly, keep you happy in life and in work.

Career Profile: Mina Ratkalkar, LCSW, M.S., Ph.D.

Where Are You Currently Working, and What Position Do You Hold?

I am currently working for myself at my private practice in Durham, North Carolina. I am the practice owner and founder. I just hired a second forensic psychologist to work with me, as the business has expanded. Recently, I began a part-time contract position at a state hospital in North Carolina conducting court-ordered capacity evaluations. There was an immediate need for forensic psychologists, and it gives me the opportunity to do some meaningful work in the public sector while continuing to work for myself.

My practice is a mix of the following:

- *Therapy for individuals, couples, and people with diverse relationship structures.* I specialize and have certification in sex therapy, but my clients do not strictly come for sex therapy. Instead, with almost every client regardless of why they're seeing me, I open the door to speaking about sexuality if they choose. When I ask these questions, people often have something meaningful to share and express gratitude to have a space to talk about something so potentially difficult and personal.
- *Treatment approaches that focus on EBPs like acceptance and commitment therapy (ACT), cognitive behavioral therapy (CBT), or integrative behavioral couple therapy for couples.* But I work with a diverse group of people of different SES. I make sure to consider people's identities in therapy and evaluation.
- *Forensic evaluation for criminal, civil, and family law cases.* I work part-time at the state hospital and also receive referrals from attorneys in my private practice. I do not do custody evaluations for family law, but I do evaluate people who want to adopt children or people interested in working with/being a gestational carrier or gamete donor.
- *Clinical supervision.* I supervise social workers working toward their LCSW, psychology interns, and undergraduate interns from UNC. I get to use both my social work and psychology training which gives me appreciation for both disciplines and their differences.
- *Speaking/trainings.* I give talks at local universities, organizations, or businesses on clinical and forensic topics. It's a wide range. If I think I can accommodate a request, I try to. But I will turn down things that are outside my scope.
- *Research.* I collaborate with academics. I am currently participating in research teams looking at ways to systemically conduct culturally responsive forensic evaluation.

I practice primarily with my psychology license in NC, but I maintain social work licenses in North Carolina, Pennsylvania, and Florida. I'm also licensed in Hawaii and through PsyPact to do clinical and forensic work with people across the country.

What Got You Interested in a Career in Working in Private-Sector Clinical Practice?

I have varied interests and multiple specialties. I was initially searching for a job that was a perfect fit, but not too many people were looking for a sex therapist AND a forensic psychologist in a job description. I did not want to have to choose between multiple types of practice that I love. I was drawn to the flexibility and truly getting to personalize what I want to do. As I learn more about the options within our field, I realize there is still much that I don't know.

I felt more certain I wanted to pursue private practice once I identified ways I could be financially comfortable in the private sector while still doing some work for underserved people.

What Does an Average Workday Look Like for You, in Terms of Duties and Responsibilities?

Some days are strictly for evaluation. Those days are spent evaluating people in jails, at the state hospital, in my office, or virtually; scoring and writing assessments; etc. More often, I have a mix of therapy and evaluation clients in the same day. I typically examine my schedule for the day, see which types of therapy or resources I need for my clients, and gather those (e.g., specific worksheets or workbooks, a recommendation I want to give, etc.) I have worked on making documentation simultaneous using an e-ink notebook, so I rarely have clinical notes to do after therapy sessions anymore. I realized I do better when I have blocks of time set aside rather than jumping from therapy to evaluation hour by hour. So I try to block two to three hours at a time for writing, collateral calls for an evaluation, record review, etc. Also, as a business owner, I have a lot of administrative duties to manage. So I try to block one day a week for about three hours for administrative work (talking to my bookkeeper, purchasing testing, invoicing, etc.). I hired a virtual assistant early to help with those tasks since I knew I would not be able to keep up with everything on my own. I outsourced scheduling as much as possible.

What Is the Most Rewarding Aspect of Your Work?

I love seeing clients reach their therapy goals or find more meaning in their relationships.

Through some referral sources, I get to see people who could typically never afford private practice therapy. I wake up excited to go to work most days, and I never take that for granted.

Sex therapy is particularly rewarding. Though some of the topics are serious (i.e., sexual assault), I often get to laugh with clients and use humor to navigate the inherent awkwardness of some conversations related to sexuality. There is also typically a big psychoeducation component since sex ed is very lacking in most places, and information people find online can be a mixed bag.

With the forensic side, I love the intellectual stimulation of it and try to work on different types of cases. Working with interns and more recent psychology graduates is particularly rewarding. I learn so much by supervising, and I have more reflective practice because of the opportunity. I also get to teach students this way without having an academic position.

With interns from local universities, I get access to resources like library access and literature review. I also love opportunities to testify on specific topics rather than doing strictly evaluations. For example, I testified in Colorado specifically on consent as an expert witness.

I also keep finding things within psychology that I want to explore. Currently, I'm working with a colleague on developing groups for adults with ADHD and workshops on considering neurodiversity in intimacy. Creative work like this with a real human impact makes me happy. I appreciate working with interdisciplinary teams and consult with lawyers, doctors, occupational therapists, computer scientists, etc., about different ideas outside the typical scope of a psychological practice (e.g., ways to use VR to help people improve their social skills, recommendations for products for neurodiverse clients who want to optimize their workspace, innovations in sexual and reproductive health).

What Have Been Some of the Most Challenging Things to Navigate in Your Work?

The sheer amount of administrative responsibilities and processes needed for compliance (i.e., annual forms for business and professional licensing) is daunting. Even in hiring in-person and virtual assistants, I can be a bottleneck because they wait on my responses. I learned that delegating entire responsibilities rather than specific tasks is more helpful. For example, I hired a bookkeeper and accountant, and I ask my office manager to send them information they need regularly. Of course, I keep an eye on my own finances, but hiring other people to do things more efficiently and consistently has been money well spent. Some referral sources do not pay until after work is done, and that can be challenging. I work with adults, and many couples want to meet after business hours. I don't mind working at night, but it does make it tougher to connect with my partner or family since I'm working sometimes when they're free.

Because I do so many different things in my practice, I must be deliberate about considering the mental and time cost of task switching. Ideally, I'd time block my day by type of task (writing, admin/phone calls). In reality, I might have to squeeze in a therapy client, review records quickly, and answer people who are waiting on my responses before moving forward with different projects. Additionally, the flexibility of private practice has made it easy for me to say yes to too many things, like seeing clients outside of hours I initially said I wouldn't. The different ideas I have for workshops, e-books, etc., do not pay off if I abandon the project when something more interesting comes along. I've learned to write down ideas and think about them more sincerely before committing. AI has been helpful with this to get rid of the "blank page" problem.

If Someone Wanted to Follow in Your Footsteps, What Advice Would You Give Them?

For anyone who is vaguely interested in sex therapy or forensic psychology, do it! Ask widely for mentorship. It does not need to be from a well-established professional, necessarily. I have found it helpful to speak to people just a couple of years ahead of where I am, as well as people decades into a successful career. Also, getting involved early in organizations like American Association of Sexuality Educators (for sex therapy) or American Academy of Forensic Psychology (for forensic psychology) was helpful. Start small with a private practice (a few clients a week part time) if you are financially worried about going out on your own full-time. Get a good lawyer, accountant, malpractice insurance, and bookkeeper/bookkeeping software right away to make sure your business structure is sound. If you must get your own benefits like I did, shop around and plan for things like potential disabilities or a dental emergency. Do not be shy about charging for your services. There are plenty of people or organizations who can pay full fee, and you can always have sliding scale or *pro bono* services for those who can't.

Consider whether you are someone who appreciates routine or someone who values flexibility. Create the practice that works for YOU, your schedule, and your family. Expect to make mistakes. I learned over time that keeping fairly set hours works best for me, but I make sure to take advantage of the flexibility I created—like running errands or paddleboarding during typical American work hours—to remind myself that the stress of running a business is well worth it.

REFERENCES

Archer, R. P., Wheeler, M. A., & Vauter, R. A. (2016). Empirically supported forensic assessment. *Clinical Psychology: Science and Practice, 23*(4), 348–364. https://doi.org/10.1111/cpsp.12171

Clay, R. A. (2009). Postgrad growth area: Forensic psychology. *gradPSYCH Magazine, 7*(4), 11. https://www.apa.org/gradpsych/2009/11/postgrad

Cox, J., Stinar, L. D., & Foster, E. E. (2017). On being a novice forensic evaluator: Reflections from early career forensic psychologists. *Psychological Injury and Law, 10*(2), 191–195. https://doi.org/10.1007/s12207-017-9281-y

DeMatteo, D., Fairfax-Columbo, J., & Desai, A. (2020). *Becoming a forensic psychologist.* Routledge.

Federal Rules of Civil Procedure. (2024). U.S. Government Publishing Office. https://www.uscourts.gov/sites/default/files/civil_federal_rules_pamphlet_dec_1_2023.pdf

Guarnera, L. A., Murrie, D. C., & Boccaccini, M. T. (2017). Why do forensic experts disagree? Sources of unreliability and bias in forensic psychology evaluations. *Translational Issues in Psychological Science, 3*(2), 143–152. https://doi.org/10.1037/tps0000114

Habben, C. J. (2005). Group practice adapting private practice to the new marketplace. In R. D. Morgan, T. L. Kuther, & C. J. Habben (Eds.), *Life after graduate school in psychology: Insider's advice from new psychologists* (pp. 96–112). Psychology Press.

Heilbrun, K. (2001). *Principles of forensic mental health assessment*. Kluwer Academic/Plenum Publishers.

LaDuke, C., DeMatteo, D., Brank, E. M., & Kavanaugh, A. (2024). Training, practice, and career considerations in forensic psychology: Results from a field survey of clinical and non-clinical professionals in the United States. *Frontiers in Psychology, 15*, 1439874. https://doi.org/10.3389/fpsyg.2024.1439874

Mart, E. (2006). *Getting started in forensic psychology practice: How to create a forensic specialty in your mental health practice*. John Wiley & Sons.

Mart, E. (2007). Growing your forensic practice. *The Journal of Psychiatry & Law, 35*(2), 147–171. https://doi.org/10.1177/009318530703500204

Melton, G. B., Petrila, J., Poythress, N. G., Slobogin, C., Otto, R. K., Mossman, D., & Condie, L. O. (2018). *Psychological evaluations for the courts: A handbook for mental health professionals and lawyers* (4th ed.). The Guilford Press.

Murrie, D. C., & Boccaccini, M. T. (2015). Adversarial allegiance among expert witnesses. *Annual Review of Law and Social Science, 11*, 37–55. https://doi.org/10.1146/annurev-lawsocsci-120814-121714

Neal, T. M. S., & Line, E. N. (2022). Income, demographics, and life experiences of clinical-forensic psychologists in the United States. *Frontiers in Psychology, 13*, 910672. https://doi.org/10.3389/fpsyg.2022.910672

Neal, T. M. S., Martire, K. A., Johan, J. L., Mathers, E. M., & Otto, R. K. (2022). The law meets psychological expertise: Eight best practices to improve forensic psychological assessment. *Annual Review of Law and Social Science, 18*, 169–192. https://doi.org/10.1146/annurev-lawsocsci-050420-010148

Neal, T. M. S., Slobogin, C., Saks, M. J., Faigman, D. L., & Geisinger, K. F. (2019). Psychological assessment in legal contexts: Are courts keeping "junk science" out of the courtroom? *Psychological Science in the Public Interest, 20*(3), 135–164. https://doi.org/10.1177/1529100619888860

Otto, R. K., DeMier, R. T., & Boccaccini, M. T. (2014). *Forensic reports & testimony: A guide to effective communication for psychologists & psychiatrists*. John Wiley & Sons.

Thompson, D. W., & Frumkin, I. (2023). Recommendations for establishing or expanding a successful forensic psychology practice. *Practice Innovations, 8*(3), 209–220. https://doi.org/10.1037/pri0000203

Vineberg, D. (2005). Independent practice alive or dead? In R. D. Morgan, T. L. Kuther, & C. J. Habben (Eds.), *Life after graduate school in psychology: Insider's advice from new psychologists* (pp. 86–96). Psychology Press.

Zapf, P. A., & Dror, I. E. (2017). Understanding and mitigating bias in forensic evaluation: Lessons from forensic science. *The International Journal of Forensic Mental Health, 16*(3), 227–238. https://doi.org/10.1080/14999013.2017.1317302

Part IV

Accomplishing Systems-Level Change

An Exploration of Policy Work in Forensic Psychology

CHAPTER 8

I Want a Pension!

Doing Policy Work Via Government Agencies

As we've mentioned earlier in this book, forensic psychologists leverage their expertise in the mental health, civil, and criminal justice systems to influence policy. Roles within the government provide one such avenue for this impact. The American system of government disperses power between the federal government and the state governments, each consisting of three branches. Within each branch are various government departments organized into agencies, bureaus, divisions, and offices, each with different authority over public policy. Forensic psychologists can influence public policy at all levels of the government—county, state, and federal—via relevant mental health, civil, and criminal justice agencies. These agencies function as the strategic players behind the scenes, identifying gaps in the system, conducting innovative research, and implementing new practices. The scope of possibilities is so expansive that it would be impossible to list them all in one chapter. Instead, we delve into several examples that showcase how government agencies have played pivotal roles in policy changes pertaining to forensic psychology. We hope to get your wheels turning as to how you can contribute to shaping laws, policies, and practices that impact individuals with mental health needs and justice involvement.

THERAPEUTIC JURISPRUDENCE

Several theoretical foundations underpin the intersection of psychological principles and the law and are paramount to influencing forensic mental health policy. Laws are formed with the underlying assumption that they will influence human behavior. For example, criminal sanctions are based on

DOI: 10.4324/9781003408857-12

the belief that the threat of punishment will deter individuals from engaging in specific behavior or to exact retribution for undesirable and harmful behavior. However, another key principle of punishment is that of *rehabilitation*. *Therapeutic jurisprudence* represents a rehabilitative framework that emphasizes the law's ability to help benefit an individual's psychological state and well-being (Wexler & Winick, 1991). It aims to maximize the therapeutic while minimizing the nontherapeutic effects of the law. For example, therapeutic jurisprudence has been applied to advanced directives, a legal document in which individuals can state their treatment preferences in the event that they become incapacitated. These documents protect individual's autonomy and ability to direct their own care in a crisis situation (SAMHSA, 2019a). This approach also includes examining the impact of the law on defendants or victims, which encompasses the effect of specific laws, the procedures of the justice system, and the roles of legal players (e.g., judges, law enforcement, lawyers) (American Psychological Association, 2018; Winick, 2006).

The therapeutic jurisprudence framework is pivotal to forensic psychology, as it identifies areas of the law to which to apply principles of psychology. For example, individuals with mental health disorders have specific treatment needs that are unmet in the standard model of prosecution (e.g., incarceration). A therapeutic jurisprudence lens would suggest an alternative to incarceration, such as a diversion program, to promote well-being and treatment. Over the years, this framework has uncovered aspects of the law in need of critical examination and, in many cases, reform. This work has dramatically impacted many aspects of the law, resulting in new and innovative programs, policies, processes, and legislation.

INFLUENCING POLICY

Shaping policy is a gradual process that typically involves multiple actions rather than a quick, one-step approach. Although patience is vital for the slow-moving and bureaucratic cogs of the government, the efforts invested in each stage of policy reform can lead to meaningful change.

Formation of Policy

Public policies are formed and adopted across the branches and agencies of government. In the case of legislation, regulation, litigation, and executive orders, they are legally binding. In other cases, policies may serve as mandates but may also serve as guidance for action (Pollack Porter et al., 2018). The policymaking process involves identifying a problem, proposing targeted solutions, and achieving the necessary political support to dedicate time and resources to the topic and solution (Guerrero et al., 2019).

Implementation of Policy

Developing a new policy marks the beginning of the process, as the policy must be implemented into practice. Much of the policy's success or failure hinges on the ability of the governing agency to implement it effectively. This work includes making minor or major updates to existing policies and allocating resources, such as finances and personnel (Pollack Porter et al., 2018).

Evaluation of Policy

Existing policies must be evaluated to assess their content, implementation, and impact. This aspect of policy focuses on practical impact and helps determine whether a policy effectively addresses its intended purpose. Policy evaluation creates a cyclical policymaking process, as it uncovers whether the policy was effective. If the policy is effective, then this may lead to the expansion of the policy to other areas of government or broader practice. If the policy is ineffective, it may lead to the revision of the policy, or it may lead to the elimination of the policy and the implementation of new policies that might better accomplish outcomes of interest (Centers for Disease Control and Prevention, 2014).

Affecting policy change is a nonlinear process and often involves collaborative efforts across multiple systems. Rarely does one singular entity have sole influence over shaping a policy; instead, organizations work together to influence policy and create meaningful change. In many cases, policy reform in forensic mental health has been adopted with community agency participation, which grew to eventually inspire government action.

A salient example comes from the drug court movement. In the late 1980s, Miami-Dade County, Florida, pioneered the establishment of the first drug court in the United States (Office of Justice Programs, 2023). Local authorities recognized the ineffectiveness of standard prosecution for decreasing drug use or drug-related crimes and believed that community-based interventions would better target treatment needs. The program's effective implementation involved collaboration among the local criminal justice agencies, courts, and community-based treatment centers. Further, there was a need for education and training, funding to maintain the court, and ongoing evaluation to determine if the program was successful, with additional agencies contributing to each area. Over the following years, drug courts expanded rapidly to other county and state jurisdictions, as well as received support via federal legislation. As of 2024, over 4,000 drug treatment courts exist, supported by local, state, and federal funding. Further, the effectiveness of drug courts led to the creation of other types of problem-solving courts, such as mental health courts (DeMatteo et al., 2019; National Institute of Justice, 1995; Office of Justice Programs, 2023).

GOVERNMENT AGENCIES AT THE INTERSECTION OF PSYCHOLOGY AND LAW

In the United States, the Executive Branch of the government is organized bureaucratically. This means that the responsibility for implementing and executing policy is designated to specific specialty departments and their subordinate entities. For example, the Department of Justice oversees the enforcement of federal laws. It is divided into over 40 subordinate agencies, each with a specific mission and designated role. State and county governments are structured similarly, with each locality having a structure and scope of influence.

A SYMBIOTIC RELATIONSHIP: NON-PROFITS AND GOVERNMENT

As you'll read about in Chapter 9, another common path for influencing policy is via a non-profit agency. Often, governments and non-profits collaborate, such as using public funding and resources to facilitate non-profits in delivering treatment services or non-profits conducting research on government programmatic outcomes.

This section will explore examples of governmental agencies and departments and specific examples of programs that have contributed to systems-level change. As we mentioned earlier, policy change often includes the work of multiple agencies and levels of government. Programs are listed under one specific organization or agency, but keep in mind the additional players that contributed to developing the program into what it is today. This list is by no means comprehensive but rather is merely a handful of the agencies, entities, and programs that shape the forensic mental health system.

The Criminal Justice System

Many agencies comprise the United States criminal justice system, encompassing the police, courts, and corrections. Additionally, specific agencies support the criminal justice system through research, training, grant administration, and policy development and implementation.

The Bureau of Justice Administration

The Bureau of Justice Administration (BJA) is a federal agency within the Department of Justice that focuses on policy efforts to promote reform in the criminal justice system. BJA provides training, resources, and technical assistance across the full range of agencies that have contact with justice-involved individuals (Bureau of Justice Administration, 2022). One notable initiative is the Justice and Mental Health Collaboration Program (JMHCP). This program provides grants to states, local governments, and federally recognized tribal nations for cross-system collaboration between the criminal justice and mental health system. JMHCP grants, along with other BJA grants, have been instrumental in advancing initiatives that embrace a rehabilitative and therapeutic jurisprudence approach, such as the following: crisis services, partnerships between law enforcement and mental health services, mental health diversion, in-reach (i.e., prerelease) services for community-based behavioral health providers, and mental health reentry programs (Justice Center, 2023).

Bureau of Prisons

Another notable federal agency within the Department of Justice is the Bureau of Prisons (BOP), which oversees the care and detention of all federal correctional settings and incarcerated individuals. The National Institute of Corrections is housed within the BOP, which advances policy in correctional settings at all levels through training, technical assistance, support for research, and implementation of promising practices. Additionally, the BOP contributes to developing new treatment programs for individuals with behavioral health needs. For example, the Residential Drug Abuse Program applies a therapeutic community model to address substance use disorders in federal correctional settings. Individuals in the program participate in intensive daily programming and are housed in a separate unit from the general population. These programs are widely implemented, with multiple federal correctional institutions hosting them (Bureau of Prisons, n.d.)

Problem-Solving Courts

As mentioned earlier in this chapter, problem-solving courts, such as drug courts, have impacted the forensic behavioral health policy landscape (see DeMatteo et al., 2019, for a comprehensive review). These programs were some of the early shifts toward a rehabilitative approach for individuals with behavioral health needs to address their overrepresentation in the criminal justice system. Generally, problem-solving courts aim to address the underlying factors contributing to an individual's criminal behavior, focusing on a particular population. In addition to drug courts, problem-solving courts include mental health courts, domestic violence courts, veteran's courts, and reentry courts, among others. To successfully operate, the courts require buy-in from the jurisdiction's criminal justice system stakeholders and mental health providers. Although the courts typically operate at the county level, much of the funding for operations and research comes from federal and state budgets or grants.

Law Enforcement

Law enforcement is an individual's first point of contact with the criminal justice system, presenting an opportunity for implementing deflection (police-assisted diversion) policies. An influx of mental health-related police calls that frequently result in negative outcomes has contributed to increased awareness of the need for programs to improve law enforcement responses to individuals with mental health and substance use disorders. Programs have focused on improving training for police response to crisis calls and co-response models, responding with both police and mental health clinicians (Marcus & Stergiopoulos, 2022).

Law Enforcement Assisted Diversion (LEAD) is one program that uses a harm reduction approach to divert individuals from the criminal justice system to the behavioral healthcare system. The program was first piloted in 2011 in Seattle, Washington, focusing specifically on individuals with low-level drug and prostitution offenses. Program participants are deflected before booking and connected to harm reduction case management services. The program collaborates with clients to engage them with community services, such as housing, medical care, legal assistance, job training, mental health treatment, and substance use treatment (Collins et al., 2017). LEAD has gained substantial traction, extending its reach to cities throughout the United States. Each location has fostered collaboration between local law enforcement, prosecutors, defense attorneys, treatment personnel, and individuals with behavioral health and substance use challenges (Center for Police Research and Policy, 2021).

Mental Health Agencies

A wide variety of government agencies address mental health in the United States. Federally, they include administrative agencies that support treatment services through conducting research, regulating and creating policies, administrating resources, and leading national public health initiatives. The federal government also oversees the Department of Veterans Affairs, which delivers healthcare to veterans. Much of the decision making power in mental health services falls onto the state and county, which operate mental health services and allocate funds to community providers.

State Mental Health Agencies (SMHA)

Each state has a mental health agency that organizes, finances, and delivers mental health services. States oversee both community-based mental health services and forensic and psychiatric inpatient facilities. Additionally, they provide services for individuals with justice involvement, either as the sole provider or in collaboration with the state's Department of Corrections. In many states, they conduct forensic mental health evaluations for the courts, and the majority of SMHAs share responsibility for the administration of mental health services in correctional settings.

FORENSIC (NOT SO FUN) FACT

Deinstitutionalization first began in the mid-20th century to transition individuals with severe mental illness out of psychiatric hospitals and into community treatment settings. Most states quickly joined the trend, drastically cutting inpatient beds. Although there are strategies to intercept these individuals prior to needing hospitalization, many individuals with serious mental illness languish in correctional settings and emergency departments waiting to receive needed treatment (Fuller Torrey, 2015).

The vast majority of SMHAs are responsible for delivering treatment to justice-involved individuals who meet the criteria for psychiatric hospitalization. These individuals are often transferred to state psychiatric hospitals for reasons such as incompetence to stand trial, not guilty by reason of insanity, awaiting pretrial psychological evaluations, and civilly committed sex offenders (Substance Abuse and Mental Health Services Administration, 2017). However, deinstitutionalization has resulted in a shortage of beds in state hospitals, and states are beginning to focus on policy reform to address the influx of individuals with serious mental illness into forensic settings. Examples of strategies include conducting competency evaluations and restoration in the community and jails; monitoring and tracking hospital bed waitlists and competency restoration program outcomes; and considering differences among populations, such as juveniles, individuals with intellectual disabilities, and those with cognitive deficits (Fuller Torrey, 2015; Heilbrun et al., 2019).

Substance Abuse and Mental Health Services Administration

The Substance Abuse and Mental Health Services Administration (SAMHSA) is a federal agency within the Department of Health and Human Services. SAMHSA does not directly provide mental health and substance abuse services. Instead, it supports community treatment by administering grants, providing technical assistance, and conducting research for programs related to prevention, early intervention, treatment, and education and training. Funding is available to states, communities, tribes, education agencies, and local organizations. Additionally, the agency guides the development and implementation of evidence-based practices through publishing toolkits, resource guides, and supporting program evaluations (Duff, 2020).

SAMHSA is integrally involved in facilitating treatment across the justice system for individuals with behavioral health needs. The Gather, Assess, Integrate, Network, and Stimulate (GAINS) Center provides technical assistance to expand and support community services for justice-involved individuals with behavioral health disorders. Initiatives additionally focus on cross-system training and collaboration (SAMHSA, 2022). For example, they train and educate criminal justice personnel, such as law enforcement and probation officers. This training provides them with tools to screen and identify individuals with behavioral health disorders and divert them to community treatment. Simultaneously, they support training behavioral health professionals on the criminal justice system and criminogenic risk to ensure individuals are matched to the appropriate level of services based on the principles of the risk-need-responsivity model (SAMHSA, 2019b).

KNOW THE LINGO!

The risk-need-responsivity model guides individualized treatment planning and delivery for justice-involved individuals. The approach emphasizes matching intensity of intervention to the individual's level of risk, targeting criminogenic needs, and tailoring the delivery of services to the individual's capacities and circumstances (Bonta & Andrews, 2023).

The National Institute of Mental Health

The National Institute of Mental Health (NIMH) is a federal agency housed within the National Institutes of Health that conducts research regarding mental health disorders. Both agencies support basic, clinical, and translational research externally through providing grant funding and internal laboratories. As leaders in funding behavioral health research, the research priorities of NIMH shape the direction of the field.

Stepping Up (www.stepuptogether.org) is one forensic mental health policy initiative NIMH supports with research funding. Stepping Up is a national effort to reduce the over-incarceration of individuals with behavioral health disorders through diversion to community treatment. Several organizations, including the Council for State Governments, the National Association of Counties, and the American Psychiatric Foundation, lead the initiative. The NIMH has supported Stepping Up with over 3.5 million dollars of research funding (NIMH, 2020).

United States Department of Veterans Affairs

The United States Department of Veterans Affairs (VA) provides healthcare for Veterans in the United States, operating the nation's largest integrated healthcare network (U.S. Department of Veterans Affairs, 2023). The Office of Mental Health and Suicide Prevention (OMHSP) supports the VA's delivery of evidence-based treatments, including crisis care, overdose prevention, and a wide variety of inpatient and outpatient programs. Many veterans have histories of justice involvement. Though not directly involved in diversionary processes, Veterans Justice Programs often serves as a liaison to treatment for justice-involved veterans. Outreach focuses on identifying veterans at all points of contact in the system to engage them in VA benefits, such as mental health and substance use services. Additionally, mental health social workers, psychologists, and addiction clinicians work with the courts and jails to provide transition planning and connection to services upon reentry (Blue-Howells et al., 2013).

CHAPTER TAKEAWAYS

The opportunities for shaping policy at the intersection of psychology and the law from within government agencies are vast, spanning the various sectors of the government. In this chapter, we provided specific instances of these government agencies spanning both the criminal justice and mental health systems, as well as the policies they were instrumental in developing.

With growing demand and attention for reform in both the mental health and justice systems, we anticipate a rapid and increasing impact from these agencies.

Career Profile: Matthew Stimmel, Ph.D.

Where Are You Currently Working, and What Position Do You Hold?

I currently work for the United States Department of Veterans Affairs in the Homeless Programs Office (HPO). I am the National Training Director for Veterans Justice Programs (VJP) within HPO. My main responsibility is to develop and sustain education and training for more than 550 VJP staff throughout VA Medical Centers across the country. VJP staff contribute to national policy on veterans' legal system involvement and cultivate operational partnerships to advance VJP's mission to provide access and care to veterans dealing with legal involvement, reducing their risk of recidivism, homelessness, and other adverse events, including overdose and suicide.

I am also a clinical assistant professor affiliated with the Stanford University School of Medicine, Department of Psychiatry.

What Got You Interested in a Career in Working in Public Sector Practice and Government Policy Work?

I always had an interest in public sector psychology, as both of my parents worked in healthcare and dedicated part, or all, of their careers to public service. I was a graduate student during the wars in Iraq and Afghanistan and could not help but be aware of the increasing reports of veterans returning from deployments with significant incidences of posttraumatic stress disorder (PTSD), traumatic brain injury (TBI), and substance use disorders, among other physical and mental health injuries. At the time, my research focused on trauma, while my main clinical work was in forensic settings. Although I felt a strong sense of obligation toward supporting veterans returning from deployments and separating from their service, I was unsure of how to combine these different threads of clinical interest, social justice, and public service.

During my pre-doctoral forensic psychology internship at the University of Massachusetts, I sought mentorship from a psychologist who worked at both UMass and the Bedford VA Medical Center. It was through my work with Dr. Smelson that I became aware of VJP and its robust history at the VA Palo Alto Health Care System. So I went to VA Palo Alto for my postdoctoral fellowship in their trauma emphasis area and immediately called up their local VJP supervisor to learn how I could get involved in serving veterans with criminal legal involvement. From there, I was lucky enough to get hired as a VJP Specialist, traveling to jails and courts across Northern California assisting veterans with getting access to VA services rather than continuing a carceral path in response to their legal involvement. I also collaborated with community partners to establish Veterans Treatment Courts, co-responding teams, and other innovative responses to the unique needs of veterans with legal involvement across the sequential intercept model.

What Does an Average Workday Look Like for You, in Terms of Duties and Responsibilities?

As a VJP specialist, I worked in direct veteran care and had a rotating schedule traveling to various county jails and Veteran Treatment Courts to assess veterans and support their treatment needs. I also regularly provided training on veteran-specific issues, including military culture, PTSD, TBI, and crisis intervention to community providers across the legal system spectrum, i.e., police, probation, bar associations, and veterans service organizations.

My current role is administrative, so my focus on support and advocacy has shifted from veterans to our terrific and dedicated team of VJP staff. These are primarily social workers but also psychologists, licensed counselors, and peer specialists, who are working in more than 2,000 jails, 1,000 prisons, and 700 Veterans Treatment Courts across the country. In this role, I develop all our training and educational offerings. This includes weekly and monthly consultation and training calls, annual training conferences, and partnering with other VA program offices on content development focused on veterans with legal system involvement.

I also am a member of several Homeless Programs Office working committees, including the Racial Equity and Racial Justice Workgroup, the Homeless Learning Advisory Committee, the Trauma Informed Care Dissemination Committee, the Clinical Services' DEI Workgroup, HPO Strategic Planning Committee, and Anti-Human Trafficking pilot program advisory committee. All of these aim to enhance the care and experience of veterans and staff alike within homeless programs, including VJP, and VA more generally.

Both in my direct role within VJP and as a member of these committees, I work with numerous internal and external partners, including federal and local government agencies, non-profits, and veterans advocacy groups.

What Is the Most Rewarding Aspect of Your Work?

The most rewarding aspect of my job is working directly with healthcare professionals, who share the value of service and are tirelessly dedicated to helping veterans, especially those with legal system involvement. Having been a VJP specialist myself, I know how difficult it is to spend time away on the road and working in jails and prisons, how hard it is to straddle between and advocate within large legal and healthcare systems over which you have no control, and how challenging it can be despite that to persevere and still find ways to influence systems change that can support veterans' recovery and improve their long-term health. As such, every time I can help a VJP staff member resolve a challenge, make their job easier through providing internal advocacy, or make them feel more confident in their job by providing education and training, I feel the rewards of my job, as it results in a direct change in the provided care.

Perhaps the most fun I have is during our weekly "office hours," a 60-minute consultation call I host every Thursday when staff members share the incredible success stories of the veterans they've helped—whether it's resolving a legal issue, reuniting with family, graduating from school, finding a job, or celebrating recovery. I am immensely proud of our staff and their hard work.

What Have Been Some of the Most Challenging Things to Navigate in Your Work?

I think the hardest part of working in the public sector is that you are subject to the systems you work in. I love the VA and know it provides incredible care. It is also a massive healthcare system, navigating through which can feel overwhelming at times.

Similarly, we work directly with many local, state, and federal legal systems and governmental partners, and those systems have their structures and barriers that can make it difficult to effectively support veterans in the way we would like. Although the complexity of both legal and healthcare systems can be overwhelming, familiarity with both can also sometimes provide a deeper understanding how to advocate for veterans within each. And I firmly believe that both within VA and with our external partners, we all share the same mission of serving veterans, despite how these respective systems are built making it challenging at times to accomplish that mission.

If Someone Wanted to Follow in Your Footsteps, What Advice Would You Give Them?

Stay creative! First, one of the wonderful things about being a clinical psychologist is the multiple professional paths your career can take. At times, it can feel impossible to find a direction encompassing all your interests, but if you think creatively and leverage the mentorship and relationships you've established, you might surprise yourself.

Second, the challenges of working within rigid and overly regulated systems, especially some that are inequitable, can make it feel like your individual voice doesn't matter or that established rules remain and there is no way to initiate change. But that simply has not been my experience.

There are many dedicated people in leadership constantly thinking of ways to innovate and expand the services we provide.

Working within governmental systems involves hearing "no" a lot, but it often turns into a "yes" if you advocate for what you believe in and think outside the box. I know at VA I've felt tremendous freedom to innovate education and training programs and empower our staff to translate that into the work they provide for veterans. So stay creative, stay true to your values, stay open to opportunities that might surprise you, and have some fun along the way. Our work is hard, and the rewards are found in the care we give to it and to ourselves.

REFERENCES

American Psychological Association. (2018). Therapeutic jurisprudence. In *APA dictionary of psychology*. https://dictionary.apa.org/therapeutic-jurisprudence

Blue-Howells, J. H., Clark, S. C., van den Berk-Clark, C., & McGuire, J. F. (2013). The U.S. Department of Veterans Affairs Veterans Justice programs and the Sequential Intercept Model: Case examples in national dissemination of intervention for justice-involved veterans. *Psychological Services, 10*(1), 48–53. https://doi.org/10.1037/a0029652

Bonta, J., & Andrews, D. A. (2023). *The psychology of criminal conduct* (7th ed.). Routledge. https://doi.org/10.4324/9781003292128

Bureau of Justice Administration. (2022, February 28). *About the bureau of justice administration*. U.S. Department of Justice. https://bja.ojp.gov/about

Bureau of Prisons. (n.d.). *Substance abuse treatment*. https://www.bop.gov/inmates/custody_and_care/substance_abuse_treatment.jsp

Center for Police Research and Policy. (2021). *Assessing the impact of Law Enforcement Assisted Diversion (LEAD): A review of the research*. University of Cincinnati. https://www.informedpoliceresponses.com/_files/ugd/313296_3fe253651ac5403bb85d85550a9149fc.pdf

Centers for Disease Control and Prevention. (2014). *Using evaluation to inform CDC's policy process*. Centers for Disease Control and Prevention, U.S. Department of Health and Human Service.

Collins, S. E., Lonczak, H. S., & Clifasefi, S. L. (2017). Seattle's Law Enforcement Assisted Diversion (LEAD): Program effects on recidivism outcomes. *Evaluation and Program Planning, 64*, 49–56. https://doi.org/10.1016/j.evalprogplan.2017.05.008

DeMatteo, D., Heilbrun, K., Arnold, S., & Thornewill, A. (2019). *Problem-solving courts and the criminal justice system*. Oxford University Press.

Duff, J. H. (2020). *Substance Abuse and Mental Health Services Administration (SAMHSA): Overview of the agency and major programs* (R46426). Congressional Research Service.

Fuller Torrey, E. (2015). Deinstitutionalization and the rise of violence. *CNS Spectrums, 20*(3), 207–214. https://doi.org/10.1017/S1092852914000753

Guerrero, M., Anderson, A. J., & Jason, L. A. (2019). Public policy. In L. A. Jason, O. Glantsman, O'Brien, J. F., & K. N. Ramian (Eds.), *Introduction to community psychology* (pp. 265–285). Rebus Foundation. https://press.rebus.community/introductiontocommunitypsychology/

Heilbrun, K., Giallella, C., Wright, H. J., DeMatteo, D., Griffin, P. A., Locklair, B., & Desai, A. (2019). Treatment for restoration of competence to stand trial: Critical analysis and policy recommendations. *Psychology, Public Policy, and Law, 25*(4), 266–283. https://doi.org/10.1037/law0000210

Justice Center. (2023, September). *Justice and Mental Health Collaboration program overview*. The Council of State Governments. https://csgjusticecenter.org/publications/justice-and-mental-health-collaboration-program-overview/

Marcus, N., & Stergiopoulos, V. (2022). Re-examining mental health crisis intervention: A rapid review comparing outcomes across police, co-responder, and non-police models. Health *Social Care in the Community*, *30*, 1665–1679. https://doi.org/10.1111/hsc.13731

National Institute of Justice. (1995). *The drug court movement*. U.S. Department of Justice, Office of Justice Programs. https://www.ojp.gov/pdffiles/drgctmov.pdf

National Institute of Mental Health. (2020, February 25). *Identifying practices for reducing incarceration of those with mental illnesses—A study of "Stepping Up."* https://www.nimh.nih.gov/news/science-news/2020/identifying-practices-for-reducing-incarceration-of-those-with-mental-illnesses-a-study-of-stepping-up

Office of Justice Programs. (2023, May 16). *Drug courts*. U. S. Department of Justice. https://www.ojp.gov/feature/drug-courts/overview

Pollack Porter, K. M., Rutkow, L., & McGinty, E. E. (2018). The importance of policy change for addressing public health problems. *Public Health Reports*, *133*, 9S–14S. https://doi.org/10.1177/0033354918788880

Substance Abuse and Mental Health Services Administration. (2017). *Funding and characteristics of single state agencies for substance abuse services and state mental health agencies, 2015* (HHS Pub. No. SMA-17-5029). https://store.samhsa.gov/sites/default/files/sma17-5029.pdf

Substance Abuse and Mental Health Services Administration. (2019a). *A practical guide to psychiatric advance directives*. Center for Mental Health Services. Substance Abuse and Mental Health Services Administration. https://www.samhsa.gov/sites/default/files/practical-guide-psychiatric-advance-directives.pdf

Substance Abuse and Mental Health Services Administration. (2019b). *Screening and assessment of co-occurring disorders in the justice system* (HHS Publication No. PEP19-SCREEN-CODJS). Substance Abuse and Mental Health Services Administration. https://store.samhsa.gov/sites/default/files/pep19-screen-codjs.pdf

Substance Abuse and Mental Health Services Administration. (2022, November 17). *About the GAINS center*. Substance Abuse and Mental Health Services Administration. https://www.samhsa.gov/gains-center/about

U.S. Department of Veterans Affairs. (2023, September 20). *About the department*. https://department.va.gov/about/

Wexler, D. B., & Winick, B. J. (1991). *Essays in therapeutic jurisprudence*. Carolina Academic Press.

Winick, B. J. (2006). Therapeutic jurisprudence: Enhancing the relationship between law and psychology. In B. Brooks-Gordon & M. Freeman (Eds.), *Law and psychology: Current legal issues* (Vol. 9, pp. 30–48). Oxford University Press.

CHAPTER 9

I Want to Contribute to Systems-Level Change!

Policy Work in Non-profit Organizations

By this point in the book, you likely have a good sense of what policy work as a forensic psychologist entails. However, you may be less familiar with the focus and scope of the non-profit organizations that conduct this work. Non-profit organizations promote social causes that generate public benefit rather than focusing on generating profit for business owners and relevant parties (Heaslip, 2023). They have a specific mission, which can be as broad as mental health or as narrowly focused as wrongful convictions, and their efforts are facilitated by funding from donors and funders. Those of you who have specific areas of forensic mental health that you are most passionate about may be particularly drawn to this realm of forensic psychology.

As for the scope of non-profit organizations developing and evaluating forensic mental health policies? Spoiler alert: It is vast and ever-growing. Rather than attempting to provide a comprehensive list of non-profit organizations in this realm, we aim to present a general sense of the routes you can pursue. In this chapter, we will provide examples of organizations that are established leaders in this space and the seminal work they have produced. In doing so, we hope that you will develop your own lens through which you can survey the landscape and identify non-profit organizations that are particularly well-suited to your interests and career goals.

REHABILITATIVE MODELS AND MOVEMENTS: THE NORTH STARS OF FORENSIC MENTAL HEALTH POLICY

A number of rehabilitative models and social justice movements have guided significant criminal justice reform, and they continue to heavily influence

DOI: 10.4324/9781003408857-13

policy work at the intersection of law and mental health. Interestingly, some non-profit organizations in this space were integral in *developing* said models. But more on that later. First, we will provide a primer on the foundational models directing forensic mental health policy work: the sequential intercept model (SIM), the risk-need-responsivity (RNR) model, and harm reduction. Each of these models was developed in response to the disproportional rates of mental health disorders among justice-involved individuals, the lack of sufficient resources to meet these needs, and the belief that addressing underlying mental health and psychosocial needs reduces the likelihood of criminal behavior.

Sequential Intercept Model

Developed in the early 2000s, the sequential intercept model (SIM) established a foundation for understanding, operationalizing, and developing policies that facilitate rehabilitation within the criminal justice system (Abreu et al., 2017; Griffin et al., 2015; Munetz & Griffin, 2006). Today, the SIM identifies six points—or Intercepts—at which an individual may be at risk for interacting with or is actively interacting with the criminal justice system: Community Services (e.g., the crisis care continuum; Intercept 0), Law Enforcement (Intercept 1), Initial Court Hearings and Initial Detention (Intercept 2), Jails and Courts (Intercept 3), Reentry (reintegration into the community following incarceration; Intercept 4), and Community Corrections (i.e., parole and probation; Intercept 5) (Abreu et al., 2017; Munetz & Griffin, 2006). Regarding recovery and rehabilitation, these six Intercepts also indicate opportunities for intervention and linkage to support services to break the cycle of recidivism or reduce exposure to the justice system (Munetz & Griffin, 2006).

In the years since its inception, the SIM has been widely adopted, including its notable application to the 21st Century Cures Act. In passing the Cures Act, the United States Congress identified the SIM as a strategic planning tool that can inform community-based programming aimed at reducing justice involvement among those with mental health and substance use disorders (Abreu, 2017). The SIM continues to guide the development of forensic mental health policies nationwide. For example, Minnehaha County in South Dakota applied the SIM to its planning for community triage centers, with the aim of diverting people at risk for justice involvement to treatment (Willison et al., 2018). In Ohio, the SIM informed the statewide response to the Opioid Epidemic. Specifically, the Ohio Criminal Justice Coordinating Center of Excellence identified opportunities for screening, treatment, psychoeducation, and diversion of individuals with opioid use disorder who were at risk of overdose (Bonfine et al., 2018). As a result, the state implemented evidence-based prevention programming that incorporated risk assessments, prescription drug drop-off sites, and medication-assisted treatment (Bonfine et al., 2018). In both instances, the SIM facilitated the use of rehabilitative approaches for behaviors and behavioral health disorders that often result in criminal justice involvement.

The Risk-Need-Responsivity Model

The risk-need-responsivity (RNR) model was developed in Canada in the 1980s to guide the individualized assessment and rehabilitation of those in the criminal justice system, in contrast to preexisting "one-size-fits-all" approaches (Andrews et al., 2006). This model informs treatment planning and treatment delivery for individuals with unmet psychosocial needs that contribute to their risk of offending. Per the RNR model, matching and tailoring treatment to an individual's risk of recidivism—based on level of risk and types of risk factors—leads to meaningful reductions in interactions with the criminal justice system (Andrews et al., 2006).

The RNR model is based on three principles: risk, need, and responsivity. Per the risk principle, the "dose," or intensity, of the risk-reducing intervention should match the level of risk an individual presents (Andrews & Bonta, 2010). Accordingly, high-risk individuals should receive a higher intensity intervention, while low-risk individuals should receive lower intensity intervention. The need principle specifies that criminogenic needs should be the target of treatment. Criminogenic needs are dynamic (i.e., modifiable) risk factors that contribute to recidivism, including antisocial traits, substance use, antisocial thinking patterns, antisocial peers, family and marital strain, employment and education challenges, and problems with leisure or recreation activities (Andrews & Bonta, 2010). Finally, the responsivity principle provides guidance for how treatment should be designed and delivered. According to the concept of general responsivity, evidence-based interventions should target criminogenic needs. Per the concept of specific responsivity, risk-reducing interventions should be tailored to the individual being served; this includes considering relevant individual characteristics, such as motivation, cognitive level, learning style, culture, and psychopathology.

As noted, the RNR model often informs the development of treatment for justice-involved individuals and thus sets a foundation for program evaluation. Indeed, research supports the effectiveness of providing treatment to individuals with a high risk of recidivism (Andrews & Dowden, 2007), addressing criminogenic rather than non-criminogenic needs in treatment (Bonta & Andrews, 2023), and ensuring a high level of program adherence to the RNR model (Andrews & Dowden, 2007). The RNR model has ongoing influence and relevance today. For example, in response to overcrowding and high rates of COVID-19 virus transmission in correctional settings in 2020, the RNR model was proposed as a method to direct the release of low-risk individuals (Vose et al., 2020).

Harm Reduction

The harm reduction approach focuses on reducing negative consequences associated with mental health conditions while acknowledging the realities of those conditions, such as recurring relapse in substance use disorders (Marlatt, 1996). As applied to substance use, this approach marked a radical departure from longstanding abstinence models that emphasized the need for full sobriety to achieve recovery (Marlatt, 1996). Although at times controversial, particularly within the criminal justice system (e.g., Mitchell et al., 2016), the goal of harm reduction is to meet individuals where they currently are in their recovery. In doing so, additional harms, such as the spread of infectious disease and overdose, can be mitigated in pursuit of behavioral change (e.g., reduced substance use).

Although other topics, like psychopathy and the not guilty by reason of insanity (NGRI) legal defense, may come to mind when we first think of forensic psychology, substance use disorders (SUD) are among the most common mental health disorders among justice-involved individuals (e.g., Proctor et al., 2019). In the United States, individuals with SUD frequently interact with the justice system by nature of the criminalization of drugs and due to illegal behaviors that result from substance use (e.g., driving under the influence) and crimes committed to support substance dependence (e.g., theft). Decriminalization and legalization of some substances—harm reduction approaches in and of themselves—have become increasingly common. Despite this, SUD remains heavily overrepresented in the United States criminal justice system (Bronson et al., 2017), and harm reduction continues to play a significant role in forensic mental health policy.

Harm reduction led to the development of replacement therapies and medication-assisted treatment, such as nicotine patches to support efforts to quit smoking cigarettes and methadone for individuals with opioid use disorder (Marlatt & Witkiewitz, 2010). Additionally, needle exchange programs and overdose prevention centers (alternatively called "safe injection sites") have been implemented to reduce the likelihood of blood-borne infections (e.g., HIV, hepatitis) stemming from intravenous drug use (Marlatt & Witkiewitz, 2010; Mays & Newman, 2021). Within the criminal justice system specifically, harm reduction has influenced policies to decriminalize substance use. For example, some types of Good Samaritan Laws protect individuals who report an overdose from facing prosecution, thus promoting willingness to contact authorities and increasing the likelihood of life-saving intervention (Center for Public Health Law Research, 2021). Additionally, some law enforcement trainings teach harm reduction to encourage the deflection of people with SUD from traditional criminal justice involvement, as in the case of the Law Enforcement Assisted Diversion Program (LEAD) (LEAD National Support Bureau, 2020).

Social Justice Movements

The SIM, the RNR model, and the harm reduction approach have led to great strides in the field of forensic psychology. Nonetheless, many of the issues that inspired the development of these models are ongoing, and there is a continued need for rehabilitative policies. Social justice movements in the United States provide a glimpse into these gaps. For example, in recent years, media and grassroots movements have brought attention to fatalities and injuries resulting from emergency response calls for individuals with unmet mental health needs (Marcus & Stergiopoulos, 2022). This growing nationwide awareness has resulted in efforts to develop collaborations between law enforcement and mental health providers. Such collaborative efforts focus on rehabilitation, deflection from the criminal justice system, and provision of adequate support for both the individuals with mental health disorders and first responders (Marcus & Stergiopoulos, 2022). Co-responder teams and Crisis Intervention Team training are two of the key initiatives to result from policy work and the groundwork laid by the SIM, the RNR model, and the harm reduction approach.

Co-responder Teams

Co-responder teams pair law enforcement officers with mental health providers to respond to calls for community members in a mental health crisis. This approach leverages the skillset of both professions to provide adequate services to the individual in crisis. In doing so, co-responder teams reduce the need for emergency medical services, minimize injuries, improve relationships between community members and law enforcement, and deflect individuals from arrest and incarceration (Morabito et al., 2018).

Crisis Intervention Team Training

Crisis Intervention Team trainings often follow the "Memphis model" (Compton et al., 2008), which consists of 40 hours of training. In these trainings, law enforcement and correctional officers learn how to identify individuals with mental health needs, use verbal de-escalation skills, serve as a bridge to appropriate community resources, and collaborate with relevant parties, such as advocates and mental health providers (Marcus & Stergio-poulos, 2022).

Policy development and implementation are critical for pilot testing and the subsequent widespread adoption of novel rehabilitative programming. In addition to spotlighting the decades-long efforts of forensic psychologists, social justice movements have encouraged greater willingness from commu-nities and governments to invest in the development of mental health poli-cies and programming. Needless to say, it's an exciting time to be a forensic psychologist working in policy!

NON-PROFIT ORGANIZATIONS AT THE INTERSECTION OF PSYCHOLOGY AND LAW

Within the realm of forensic psychology, non-profit organizations can be broadly separated into those with a specific focus on psychology and law and those with a broad policy focus, with forensic mental health tracks. In this section, we will review examples of both.

Law and Mental Health-Centered Non-profit Organizations

Non-profit organizations that focus specifically on forensic mental health can be distinguished further by the presence or absence of formal affiliations. Some non-profit organizations are affiliated with or supported by a univer-sity, whereas others are standalone.

University-Affiliated Non-profit Organizations

Non-profit organizations with university affiliations are typically interdis-ciplinary. They often present opportunities for job responsibilities beyond policy work, such as teaching, mentoring, clinical work, research, and con-sultation. If our discussion of policy work is piquing your interest, but you remain passionate about teaching or delivering behavioral health treatment, this domain of the non-profit sector may be particularly appealing.

As a first example, consider the Institute of Law, Psychiatry and Public Policy (ILPPP; www.ilppp.org/), a long-standing non-profit organization affiliated with the University of Virginia. With origins in the 1970s, ILPPP was established in response to a number of critical decisions by the Supreme Court of the United States (SCOTUS) and state courts: *Jackson v. Indiana*

(1972), *Lessard v. Schmidt* (1972), *and Wyatt v. Stickney* (1972) (Bonnie et al., 2021). These decisions have resulted in notable efforts to improve services and policies at the intersection of psychology and law. Given the complex and nuanced nature of these issues, many—such as the hospitalization and rehabilitation of defendants found incompetent to stand trial—remain the focus of ongoing efforts to reform the criminal justice system.

CASE LAW REVIEW

In *Jackson v. Indiana* (1972), SCOTUS held that states are not permitted to indefinitely commit defendants who are found incompetent to stand trial. Instead, the length of commitment should be determined by the likelihood of restorability. As a result, many states turned to the field of forensic psychology to guide procedures for the evaluation and treatment of criminal defendants found incompetent to stand trial.

CASE LAW REVIEW

Lessard v. Schmidt (1972) was a groundbreaking court ruling by a federal district court in Wisconsin. The court ruled that involuntary civil commitment on the grounds of mental illness alone was unconstitutional; instead, it is necessary to demonstrate that the individual presents a danger to themselves or to others. As a result, nearly every state revised its commitment laws. Forensic psychologists may contribute to the ongoing implementation of this ruling by evaluating the dangerousness of said individuals and contributing to policies on patient rights and advocacy.

ILPPP has two primary tracks, both of which work in partnership with the Virginia Department of Behavioral Health and Developmental Services (DBHDS): (1) mental health law and policy and (2) forensic mental health and the criminal justice system. This non-profit organization has been instrumental in the development of key policies in Virginia, including the following (Bonnie et al., 2021):

- the creation and use of community-based forensic services following hospital-based evaluation.
- the protection and rights of individuals who are institutionalized and of those who receive community-based services.
- efforts to support deinstitutionalization, such as crisis services and treatment facilitation for community-based individuals with chronic behavioral health disorders.

Although the focus of this chapter is policy work, it is worth highlighting the additional opportunities available at ILPPP. In addition to the forensic mental health track's focus on clinical work and clinical training, ILPPP offers educational opportunities, such as coursework in mental health law (Bonnie et al., 2021). ILPPP staff provide clinical training in forensic evaluation to community mental health providers (Bonnie et al., 2021). Finally, within the ILPPP Forensic Clinic, clinical-forensic psychologists provide forensic evaluation services to clients and specialized training to graduate students (Bonnie et al., 2021).

CASE LAW REVIEW

In *Wyatt v. Stickney* (1972), a federal court in Alabama ruled that individuals who are involuntarily committed to state hospitals due to behavioral health disorders, including developmental disorders, have a constitutional right to treatment. This ruling was a response to the overcrowding of state hospitals in Alabama and their insufficient resources. As a result, many states significantly reformed their behavioral health systems, including allocating funding to community-based treatment, developing regulations, and supporting patient advocacy.

KNOW THE LINGO

Restorative justice aims to promote healing and rehabilitation of individuals who have committed crimes by bringing them into conversation with victims and their community. The primary focus is on the harm that was caused and what is needed to repair said harm. To do so, restorative justice approaches focus on building accountability, a clear understanding of the impact of one's actions, and a path forward (Zehr & Mika, 1997).

As a second example, the Juvenile Justice Institute (JJI), developed in 2002, is a research institute housed within the University of Nebraska Omaha's School of Criminology and Criminal Justice (www.unomaha.edu/college-of-public-affairs-and-community-service/juvenile-justice-institute/index.php). In contrast to ILPPP, JJI focuses specifically on juvenile justice. This organization conducts policy and program evaluations for state agencies, local agencies, and private organizations. Past projects have included the following (Wasserburger et al., 2021):

- evaluating data on community-based programs to determine the most effective practices, for youth, including mentoring programs for juveniles involved in the justice-system.
- facilitating restorative justice.
- examining the impact of the COVID-19 pandemic on juvenile aid programs that are sponsored by the Nebraska legislature.

Similar to other university-affiliated non-profit organizations, JJI also provides university students with opportunities for involvement in research and educational development. As such, forensic psychologists who work in this environment may be able to assume additional professional roles, such as mentoring.

As a third example, the University of Southern California (USC) Gould School of Law houses the Saks Institute for Mental Health Law, Policy, and Ethics (www.gould.usc.edu/faculty/centers/saks/). This interdisciplinary think tank focuses on research, policy reform, and advocacy at the intersection of psychiatry and law. Specifically, the institute focuses on mental health law and patient rights, including the following:

- minimizing the use of restraints in psychiatric hospitals.
- patients' right to treatment with psychotropics.
- patients' right to refuse medication.

Standalone Non-profit Organizations

In contrast to non-profits that are affiliated with universities, standalone non-profit organizations are less likely to have opportunities for job responsibilities in the undergraduate or graduate teaching and clinical realms. Nonetheless, these organizations offer rich forensic mental health policy experience.

As a first example, consider Policy Research Associates, Inc. (PRA). Policy Research Associates, Inc. (PRA) is an established non-profit organization that works at the state, local, and national levels, including with government organizations (www.prainc.com). Within an overall focus on behavioral health, PRA has a specific focus at the intersection of law and behavioral health, including criminal justice and juvenile justice. The work produced by PRA has led to tremendous gains in the field. Remember when we mentioned that a non-profit organization was part of the team that developed the sequential intercept model (SIM)? Mystery solved. Examples of other research and policy-focused work that PRA has contributed to include the following:

- conducting a national survey of United States juvenile mental health courts (Callahan et al., 2012).
- evaluating the use of sanctions and incentives in mental health courts (Callahan et al., 2013).
- evaluating the fairness of algorithmic risk assessment instruments (Zottola et al., 2022).
- evaluating and providing guidance on the use of medication-assisted treatment in the criminal justice system.
- evaluating state hospitals' management of care for individuals found incompetent to stand trial.

Beyond policy work, PRA provides technical assistance to organizations as they implement evidence-based treatments for justice-involved individuals with mental health needs. For example, in collaboration with the Substance Use and Mental Health Services Administration (SAMHSA) GAINS Center, PRA is working to expand access to community-based services for individuals with co-occurring mental health and substance use disorders across the criminal justice system. Furthermore, PRA continues to provide open-access resources on SIM and offers workshops to help teams apply this model. They provide training on additional topics, such as adolescent behavioral health training for school resource officers.

If you are eager to learn more about PRA's impactful work, then you're in luck. The organization publishes a quarterly impact report that highlights their work and primary areas of impact. This report can be found via their website (www.prainc.com).

As a second example, consider the Vera Institute of Justice, founded in 1961 to support alternatives to bail in New York City (www.vera.org). Today, this non-profit organization focuses on ending overcriminalization and mass incarceration, with a particular emphasis on supporting communities that are underserved or disproportionately negatively impacted by the criminal justice system (i.e., people of color, immigrants, those experiencing poverty). The Vera Institute works at the federal, state, and local levels to conduct research, advocacy, and policy work. Specifically, the Vera Institute develops, implements, and evaluates pilot programs and subsequently identifies successful ones to scale. Current initiatives focused on the criminal justice system include the following:

- facilitating access to college education among those who are incarcerated.
- addressing systemic racial disparities in legal decision making.
- facilitating access to housing following incarceration.
- jail decarceration (i.e., reducing the number of individuals incarcerated in jails).
- improving housing units in prison.

Non-profit Organizations With a Broad Focus on Policy

Lastly, some non-profit organizations are centered on policy broadly, with behavioral health and criminal justice as distinct focuses. As a first example, consider the RAND Corporation (RAND), one of the largest and most well-established non-profit policy organizations worldwide (www.rand.org/). RAND operates globally, with a focus on using research and analysis to improve policy and related decision making.

RAND's work at the intersection of law and mental health is housed within a few research departments and centers, including Behavioral and Policy Sciences, RAND Drug Policy Research Center, and the Institute for Civil Justice.

Uniquely, RAND employs over 1,700 staff members across more than 50 countries. With such a wide scope, it is likely to find an area that interests you as a forensic psychologist. If the policy-focused non-profit wheels have already begun turning, we recommend spending some time familiarizing yourself with the work being done across RAND via their website.

The Urban Institute provides a second example. The Urban Institute is a non-profit think tank and research organization that aims to improve the well-being of communities and families via inclusive economic growth (www.urban.org). Although it is broadly focused on policy, the Urban Institute has a specific focus area in crime, justice, and safety. Related research and program evaluation efforts have included the following:

- examining alternative crisis response services in Colorado.
- evaluating transitional housing options for individuals on probation in Arizona.
- examining drug diversion programs in Massachusetts.

Mental Health Organizations

Lastly, some of the primary mental health organizations in the nation have established criminal justice tracks for policy work. For example, the National Alliance on Mental Illness (NAMI)—the largest grassroots mental health organization in the United States—has identified many criminal justice topics as policy priorities, including the criminalization of people with mental illness, use of the death penalty, gun violence, police use of force, application of restraints and seclusion, and solitary confinement.

CHAPTER SUMMARY

By now, you have familiarized yourself with the domains in which non-profit policy work can occur, ranging from narrowly to broadly focused. However, bear in mind that many more organizations exist that may be a good fit based on your specific interests in forensic mental health policy. We encourage you to use this roadmap to guide your research into these career avenues.

CAUGHT THE NON-PROFIT BUG?

If you are eager to explore more non-profit organizations that are conducting policy work in forensic mental health, consider looking into the following (not exhaustive):

- Juvenile Law Center (www.jlc.org)
- Judge David L. Bazelon Center for Mental Health Law (www.bazelon.org)
- Center for Justice Innovation (www.innovatingjustice.org)
- Council of State Governments Justice Center (www.csgjusticecenter.org)
- National Harm Reduction Coalition (www.harmreduction.org)
- National Association of State Mental Health Program Directors' Research Institute (https://www.nasmhpd.org)
- Mental Health America (https://mhanational.org)
- The Pew Charitable Trusts Mental Health and Justice Partnerships (www.pewtrusts.org/en/projects/mental-health-and-justice-partnerships)

We hope that our discussion of policy-focused non-profit organizations presented a fresh perspective on the diverse paths a career in forensic psychology can take. As covered in this chapter, there are many non-profit organizations exploring the intersection of law and psychology. These include non-profit agencies affiliated with academic institutions; standalone non-profit agencies that have a forensic mental health focus; more generalized non-profit policy agencies that have designated forensic focus tracks; and non-profit mental health agencies that engage in some policy advocacy. Given the increased focus on and widespread awareness of challenges facing the justice system—including the disproportionate representation of those with behavioral health disorders—we can anticipate that more like-minded organizations will crop up in the coming years.

Career Profile: Stephanie Brooks Holliday, Ph.D.

Where Are You Currently Working, and What Position Do You Hold?

I am Senior Behavioral Scientist at RAND, which is a non-profit, nonpartisan research organization. As an organization, RAND aims to conduct research and analysis that improves policy and decision making. As Senior Behavioral Scientist, my role involves leading and contributing to research projects.

What Got You Interested in a Career in Working in Non-Profit Policy Work?

In between undergrad and grad school, I spent two years working as a research assistant for a health policy research organization in Washington, D.C. It was my first introduction to policy-relevant research. As an undergraduate research assistant, I had worked on studies relating to intervention development and risk assessment. But at the health policy organization, I was contributing to work such as evaluating the federal block grants that provide funding to states for substance use disorder and mental health treatment. It was my first introduction to research methods applied to policy questions but still with a focus on mental health.

While I was on my clinical internship and my postdoctoral fellowship, I decided that I wanted to pursue a research-focused career. At the time, I was open to a range of settings—academia, non-profits, and government positions. When I interviewed at RAND, though, there were a few things that I found compelling. First was the commitment to using research to address critical social issues. RAND researchers were focused not just on conducting the research but also making sure that the findings reach the hands of decision makers. Second, RAND is an incredibly interdisciplinary setting. On my criminal justice-focused projects, a typical team might include a psychologist, a criminologist, a policy researcher, an economist, a statistician, a public health researcher—or some mix of all of those disciplines. This allows research projects to draw on approaches from a range of disciplines, which can enhance the rigor of the work.

What Does an Average Workday Look Like for You, in Terms of Duties and Responsibilities?

My work is fully focused on conducting research. Most research at RAND is funded through external sources, including federal grants and contracts; state, county, and city contracts; and foundation funding, among others. I'm typically leading multiple research projects which can vary quite a bit in terms of research question, methods, and timeframe. So on a typical day, I'm usually working on tasks from multiple different projects. For example, I might be submitting a survey instrument to our IRB for review for one project, meeting with a funder for another project, developing a qualitative coding process for a third project, and writing an evaluation report summarizing findings for a fourth project. Most of my work is related to the legal system, but I also contribute to projects focused on other populations or topic areas based on my interests. Every day is a little different, and being able to work on multiple funded studies keeps the work fresh and interesting.

What Is the Most Rewarding Aspect of Your Work?

By far, the most rewarding aspect of my work is when I see findings from a study actually make an impact on policies or programs. Sometimes, this happens on a small scale—for example, a program that I'm evaluating may decide to implement the recommendations that we provided. This is gratifying because it means our work is helping to optimize the implementation or outcomes of the program and that the program finds our recommendations compelling and relevant. Other times, this happens on a large scale. For example, I had a study that estimated the proportion of the mental health population within the Los Angeles County jail system that might be appropriate for diversion to community-based services. The findings from this study were cited in subsequent policy decisions related to local resources for incarcerated individuals with mental illness. Though these were local policy decisions, the Los Angeles County jail system houses more than 15,000 people, an estimated 40% of whom have a mental health condition—meaning that these policies impact a large number of people.

I also do a lot of community-engaged research, and this is very gratifying as well. I often have the chance to partner closely with community-based organizations and providers, to engage with advisory boards, and to integrate the perspectives of people with lived experience into my work. My work setting gives researchers a lot of autonomy with respect to the methods that we choose, which has made it possible to approach research in this more equity-centered manner.

What Have Been Some of the Most Challenging Things to Navigate in Your Work?

Most research conducted in my workplace is funded extramurally—which means that a key aspect of the job is applying for funding. It can be challenging to find the right balance between leading ongoing projects and planning several months into the future.

If Someone Wanted to Follow in Your Footsteps, What Advice Would You Give Them?

In many ways, preparing for a career at a policy research organization is similar to preparing for a job in an academic setting: strong research skills are essential. However, it's also valuable to begin developing the skills to think about how research translates into policy. For example, what implications do your findings have for policy, not just for practice or future research? Who are the decision makers relevant to your research topic, and how can you get creative about dissemination to make sure your findings reach that audience? It's not always possible to gain these types of experiences during training, but when the opportunity arises, it's worth taking advantage of them. For example, it could include contributing to a webinar or writing an article focused on a practitioner or policy audience. These experiences are a way to begin sharpening these types of skills and can provide a solid foundation for career in policy research.

REFERENCES

Abreu, D. (2017, February 8). *Maximizing the Cures Act by utilizing the Sequential Intercept Model.* Policy Research Associates. https://prainc.com/curesact-sim/

Abreu, D., Parker, T. W., Noether, C. D., Steadman, H. J., & Case, B. (2017). Revising the paradigm for jail diversion for people with mental and substance use disorders: Intercept 0. *Behavioral Sciences & the Law, 35,* 1–16. https://doi.org/10.1002/bsl.2300

Andrews, D. A., & Bonta, J. (2010). Rehabilitating criminal justice policy and practice. *Psychology, Public Policy & Law, 16*(1), 39–55. https://doi.org/10.1037/a0018362

Andrews, D. A., Bonta, J., & Wormith, J. S. (2006). The recent past and near future of risk and/or need assessment. *Crime & Delinquency, 52*(1), 7–27. https://doi.org/10.1177/0011128705281756

Andrews, D. A., & Dowden, C. (2007). The risk-need-responsivity model of assessment and human service in prevention and corrections: Crime-prevent jurisprudence. *Canadian Journal of Criminology and Criminal Justice, 49,* 439–464. https://doi.org/10.3138/cjccj.49.4.439

Bonfine, N., Munetz, M. R., & Simera, R. H. (2018). Sequential intercept mapping: Developing systems-level solutions for the opioid epidemic. *Psychiatric Services, 69*(11), 1124–1126. https://doi.org/10.1176/appi.ps.201800192

Bonnie, R. J., Murrie, D. C., & Zelle, H. (2021). The University of Virginia's Institute of law, psychiatry, and public policy. In K. Heilbrun, H. J. Wright, C. Giallella, & D. DeMatteo (Eds.), *University and public behavioral health organization collaboration in justice contexts* (pp. 14–29). Oxford University Press. https://doi.org/10.1093/med-psych/9780190052850.003.0002

Bonta, J., & Andrews, D. A. (2023). *The psychology of criminal conduct* (7th ed.). Routledge.

Bronson, J., Stroop, J., Zimmer, S., & Berzofsky, M. (2017). *Drug use, dependence, and abuse among state prisoners and jail inmates, 2007–2009* (NCJ 250546). U.S. Department of Justice, Bureau of Justice Statistics. https://bjs.ojp.gov/content/pub/pdf/dudaspji0709.pdf

Callahan, L., Cocozza, J., Steadman, H. J., & Tillman, S. (2012). A national survey of U.S. juvenile mental health courts. *Psychiatric Services, 63*(2), 130–134. https://doi.org/10.1176/appi.ps.201100113

Callahan, L., Steadman, H. J., Tillman, S., & Vesselinov, R. (2013). A multi-site study of the use of sanctions and incentives in mental health courts. *Law and Human Behavior, 37*(1), 1–9. https://doi.org/10.1037/h0093989

Center for Public Health Law Research. (2021). *Good Samaritan overdose prevention laws.* Prescription Drug Abuse Policy System. https://pdaps.org/datasets/good-samaritan-overdose-laws-1501695153

Compton, M. T., Bahora, M., Watson, A. C., & Oliva, J. R. (2008). A comprehensive review of extant research on Crisis Intervention Team (CIT) programs. *The Journal of the American Academy of Psychiatry and the Law, 36*(1), 47–55.

Griffin, P. A., Munetz, M., Bonfine, N., & Kemp, K. (2015). Development of the Sequential Intercept Model: The search for a conceptual model. In P. A. Griffin, K. Heilbrun, E. P. Mulvey, D. DeMatteo, & C. A. Schubert (Eds.), *The Sequential Intercept Model: Promoting community alternatives for individuals with serious mental illness* (pp. 21–39). Oxford University Press. https://doi.org/10.1093/med:psych/9780199826759.003.0002

Heaslip, E. (2023, February 6). Nonprofit vs. not-for-profit vs. for-profit: What's the difference? *U.S. Chamber of Commerce.* https://www.uschamber.com/co/start/strategy/nonprofit-vs-not-for-profit-vs-for-profit

Jackson v. Indiana, 406 U.S. 715. (1972).

LEAD National Support Bureau. (2020). *About LEAD*. https://www.leadbureau.org/about-lead

Lessard v. Schmidt, 349 F. Supp. 1078. (E.D. Wis. 1972).

Marcus, N., & Stergiopoulos, V. (2022). Re-examining mental health crisis intervention: A rapid review comparing outcomes across police, co-responder, and non-police models. *Health & Social Care in the Community, 30*, 1665–1679. https://doi.org/10.1111/hsc.13731

Marlatt, G. A. (1996). Harm reduction: Come as you are. *Addictive Behaviors, 21*(6), 779–788. https://doi.org/10.1016/0306-4603(96)00042-1

Marlatt, G. A., & Witkiewitz, K. (2010). Update on harm-reduction policy and intervention research. *Annual Review of Clinical Psychology, 6*, 591–606. https://doi.org/10.1146/annurev.clinpsy.121208.131438

Mays, J. C., & Newman, A. (2021, November 30). Nation's first supervised drug-injection sites open in New York. *The New York Times*. https://www.nytimes.com/2021/11/30/nyregion/supervised-injection-sites-nyc.html

Mitchell, S. G., Williet, J., Monico, L. B., James, A., Rudes, D. S., Viglioni, J., Schwartz, R. P., Gordon, M. S., & Friedmann, P. D. (2016). Community correctional agents' views of medication-assisted treatment: Examining their influence on treatment referrals and community supervision practices. *Substance Abuse, 37*(1), 127–133. https://doi.org/10.1080/08897077.2015.1129389

Morabito, M. S., Savage, J., Snelder, L., & Wallace, K. (2018). Police response to people with mental illnesses in a major U.S. city: The Boston experience with the co-responder model. *Victims & Offenders, 13*(8), 1093–1105. https://doi.org/10.1080/15564886.2018.1514340

Munetz, M., & Griffin, P. A. (2006). Use of the Sequential Intercept Model as an approach to decriminalization of people with serious mental illness. *Psychiatric Services, 57*, 544–549. https://doi.org/10.1176/ps.2006.57.4.544

Proctor, S. L., Hoffmann, N. G., & Raggio, A. (2019). Prevalence of substance use disorders and psychiatric conditions among county jail inmates. *Criminal Justice and Behavior, 46*(1), 24–41. https://doi.org/10.1177/00938548187960

Vose, B., Cullen, F. T., & Lee, H. (2020). Targeted release in the COVID-19 correctional crisis: Using the RNR model to save lives. *American Journal of Criminal Justice, 45*, 769–779. https://doi.org/10.1007/s12103-020-09539-z

Wasserburger, E., Hobbs, A., & Garman, J. (2021). *The impact of COVID-19 on community-based juvenile services aid programs* (No. 28). https://digitalcommons.unomaha.edu/jjireports/28

Willison, J. B., McCoy, E. F., Vasquez-Noriega, C., Regional, T., & Parker, T. (2018). *Using the Sequential Intercept Model to guide local reform: An Innovation Fund case study*. Urban Institute. https://www.urban.org/research/publication/using-sequential-intercept-model-guide-local-reform

Wyatt v. Stickney, 325 F. Supp. 781. (M.D. Ala. 1971).

Zehr, H., & Mika, H. (1997). Fundamental concepts of restorative justice. *Contemporary Justice Review: Issues in Criminal, Social, and Restorative Justice, 1*(1), 47–56.

Zottola, S. A., Desmarais, S. L., Lowder, E. M., & Duhart Clarke, S. E. (2022). Evaluating fairness of algorithmic risk assessment instruments: The problem with forcing dichotomies. *Criminal Justice and Behavior, 49*(3), 389–410. https://doi.org/10.1177/00938548211040544

Part V

Putting It All Together

An Exploration of How to Actualize Your Career in Forensic Psychology

CHAPTER 10

Balancing Priorities

Tips for Selecting the Most Appropriate Career Setting for You

By this point in the book, you may find yourself knowing more than you ever thought you needed to about forensic psychology, from the focus of the field to professional activities and the various settings in which forensic psychologists work. Hopefully, this expanded awareness carries with it potential career opportunities you had not already considered. But as we know all too well, the flipside of having a menu of options is feeling a lack of confidence in making just one decision—the elusive "best decision." We have arrived at the paradox of choice.

Many of us who chose to pursue doctoral training have interests that span multiple domains. If we did not enter graduate school passionate about developing skills across research, clinical practice, teaching, and writing, then being expected to try our hand at each likely introduced us to new interests along the way. However, the same curiosity and motivation that spurred us to seek a breadth of opportunities during our training can become a source of stress when it comes time to pick one career setting.

So how do you make the right choice for you? In this chapter, we will zoom the forensic career path lens back out to consider what matters most to you as you make career choices. We will talk through professional considerations and those impacting our lives outside of work.

PRIORITIZING THE PROFESSIONAL

When weighing any decision, it is helpful to consider both short-term and long-term implications. Pre- and postdoctoral training often come down to putting one foot in front of the other as you work toward milestones

DOI: 10.4324/9781003408857-15

in the near future. After spending years on a largely preset path, it can be challenging to attempt to forecast what a long-term career may look like. However, we encourage you to apply this dual lens of short- and long-term goal setting to your decision making early on. Although the choices you make in your early career do not necessarily determine the rest of your career, you can lend your future self a hand by working toward a larger goal simultaneously.

One Foot in Front of the Other: Decision Making for the Short-Term

What you would like to spend the majority of your work time on is one of the most relevant factors in selecting the right career setting for you—at least in the short term. Although there is significant variety in the type of job responsibilities a forensic psychologist is suited for, they broadly fall into clinical practice, policy work, research, and teaching. The extensive training forensic psychologists undergo, including graduate coursework and research experience, a pre-doctoral internship, and (sometimes) postdoctoral fellowships often helps to narrow down these interests. You may have greater clarity in your job selection process if one of these focus areas resonates with you far more than the others. To this end, it may be useful to revisit the earlier chapters that discuss broad areas of interest and job responsibilities in forensic psychology in detail.

Forecasting the Future: Decision Making for the Long-Term

As hard as it can be to imagine after many years of increasingly specialized training, our careers can take various forms over time, and the beauty of a doctorate is that we are well-trained in several professional roles and skills. This reality makes it helpful to consider the long-term as well. When you think about longevity in the field, what appeals to you most? Where do you see yourself in five years? Fifteen? Forty? Use this self-reflection to strategize and plan out your future accordingly.

An important long-term consideration is whether you see yourself spending a career in a couple of settings or continuously looking for new opportunities. If you have difficulty answering that, your own experience leading up to this point may provide valuable insight. Clinical psychology doctoral programs consist of clinical rotations or practicum placements (Hatcher et al., 2015). Additionally, some doctoral internships are structured based on rotations, allowing you to train in a number of clinical settings. If this diversity in experience was exciting and motivating, then you may find yourself interested in pursuing different opportunities throughout your career. In contrast, if switching teams and starting anew every few months brought with it a sense of dread, then settling down may be your best bet. Those of you who plan to stick it out for the long-haul and accordingly reap the benefits of a career spent in one place may be particularly suited for a government position or a tenure-track academic role. These options may offer unique employee benefits over the long-term, such as tuition waivers for dependents in academic settings or pensions upon retiring from a government role. More on that later.

In contrast, if you are someone who continuously looks to the next thing and may even want to relocate geographically over time, then your relative prioritization likely looks different. Instead of seeking security and opportunities within a set organization over time, your approach may be more focused on striking while the iron is hot. This will be particularly true depending on your interests and experiences during training. For example, imagine you are a true research-practitioner and want to incorporate both research and clinical work into your career. If you have already built up a research portfolio during graduate school and your postdoctoral training, then you may want to maintain momentum and pursue grant funding opportunities for a number of years before leaning into your interest in pursuing a clinical private practice. Depending on your personal circumstances, early career also may be a better time to work long hours in this type of competitive research environment before transitioning into a more "traditional" 40-hour work week or a flexible work schedule.

Further, some career settings are more flexible and may offer you the ability to pursue multiple interests from one home base. For example, some academic jobs may give you substantial freedom to pursue teaching, research, clinical work, and consulting, so long as you are meeting your minimum job requirements. It is not uncommon for forensic psychologists in academic settings to teach, advise on theses and dissertations, serve on committees, conduct research, publish, maintain a small forensic evaluation practice, or provide consultation to courts and other entities. Working in private practice also offers similar flexibility to craft a more individualized job experience, as opposed to one that is dictated by an inflexible job description.

The one through line here is that professional considerations related to job selection are layered, personal, and contingent on many factors. As you mull your options over, you may consider returning to these questions: Are there one or two specific activities you want to spend most of your working hours focused on? Do you yearn for a stable, secure role after years of bouncing from one training opportunity to the next? Checking in with yourself can help to focus your efforts on what matters most to you rather than relying primarily on the career choices made by others around you.

PRIORITIZING THE PERSONAL

Work-life balance means different things to each of us and may even engender an eyeroll in its seeming impossibility. Nonetheless, the reality is that much of our life is spent at work, and work is simultaneously not the sum total of our lives. Therefore, it is important to consider factors related to your quality of life and personal circumstances when deciding upon a career setting. Although non-exhaustive, some key considerations include employee benefits for you and your family, opportunities for remote or hybrid work, room for promotion and pay increases, and professional development opportunities.

Employee Benefits

Employee benefits are the indirect benefits employers provide to support the personal well-being and professional development of their employees. Some common benefits include health insurance, retirement savings plans, life insurance, flexible spending accounts (i.e., accounts that are funded with pre-tax income to cover out-of-pocket medical expenses), tuition assistance, and paid time off for vacation and illness. Although not as common, employers may also support new parents and caregivers through family leave policies (Ramsey, 2023). In addition to financial support, these benefits offer a sense of security that can help offset the impact of many stressors in life.

Employee benefits can also extend to family members, as in the case of family coverage for health insurance plans or reimbursement for children's educational costs. Within academic settings in particular, employees may be eligible for tuition benefits for themselves and their dependents— sometimes up to full tuition! These benefits may also apply retroactively. For example, at the Veterans Health Administration, benefits like the Education Debt Reduction Program and Student Loan Repayment Program (SLRP) enable employees to apply for additional support in the form of payments from one's employer that are applied directly to their student loan debt (VA Careers, n.d.). These benefits are provided in addition to a salary and significantly offset the cost of student loan debt. Further, the Public Service Loan Forgiveness (PSLF) Program is a national offering for employees who spend 10 years (i.e., the equivalent of 120 qualifying monthly payments) working in the non-profit or government sector. Through this program, the remaining balance of Direct Loans (after 120 payments) are forgiven by the government in exchange for your service (Federal Student Aid, n.d.).

Quality of Life

Employer-sponsored benefits go a long way in providing extra security and support for the long term (e.g., retirement), the unexpected (e.g., illness), and major life events (e.g., child birth, bereavement). However, for some, it is important to consider what your work and home life look like, day in, day out. One of the major changes that we have seen in the workforce in recent years, spurred by the COVID-19 pandemic, is the increased popularity of remote or hybrid work opportunities (Parker et al., 2022). In Chapter 3, we discussed the types of settings that may be more or less suited for remote work.

Others may look for more flexible structures like compressed schedules or being able to set one's own schedule. Both may allow for greater flexibility for family care responsibilities, pursuing additional work opportunities (e.g., building a part-time private practice), or for some, simply additional days off for travel or pursuing other interests. Compressed schedules often consist of a four-day work week. For most, this means working longer (e.g., 10-hour) days, but in some cases, it can entail working fewer hours overall (Goff-Dupont, 2022). At present, compressed schedules are more likely to be found in some clinical settings or academic medical centers due to a need for additional coverage hours for patient care. Setting one's own schedule is generally a benefit of private practice work and, to an extent, academic settings.

Promotion and Pay

Although it is rare to interview for a job that ensures you a promotion after a set period of time, there are certain indicators regarding the typical path of progression. Within traditional academic or healthcare settings, a set number of job titles typically exist. Although your job responsibilities may not shift considerably without corresponding shifts in job title, your salary may increase with tenure alone. In contrast, in more corporate settings, such as non-profit organizations, there can be additional room for a number of job transitions within the same organization or opportunities to leverage your experience into a larger role at a different organization.

It can be tempting to focus solely on the salary we are offered when considering a job opportunity. However, opportunity for advancement in both pay and in duties/responsibilities can significantly change the experience of working at a particular organization. It is important to consider what sorts of additional benefits or conditions you would like to have in your career and negotiate those alongside salary negotiations. Remember, if it is not discussed in advance and not included in writing in your contract, then you cannot assume that your job circumstances will change notably once you are in the door.

Professional Development Opportunities

A final consideration in prioritizing the personal is considering a job's ability to facilitate your own professional development. This may correspond to opportunities for increased pay or expanded duties, as covered earlier. However, it also might encompass the ability to build new skills. Some jobs may allow you to cross train for other roles or attend trainings that are of professional interest to you. For example, forensic psychologists working in treatment-oriented settings might request to attend advanced training workshops on trauma-informed care or suicide prevention. Some jobs may provide professional development funds to help forensic psychologists finance continuing education credits needed to maintain their license. Some jobs might even cover costs of license renewal or of pursuing board certification! Additionally, some employers may provide funding to attend professional conferences and networking events, such as the American Psychology-Law Society Conference or the American Academy of Forensic Psychology's Annual Meeting. Further, some employers may let forensic psychologists pursue these development opportunities on company time. Though it may not seem like much, flexibility and funding to pursue professional development is not a guarantee at all jobs. As such, you may find that jobs that support this type of professional development suit your liking more than those that do not.

MYTH BUSTING: LESSONS LEARNED FROM OUR EVOLVING CAREERS

Recommendations for professional and personal factors abound when considering a career path. But ultimately, they are unique to you and your circumstances. So we thought it would be helpful to focus on the overarching messages that a clearly laid-out career roadmap may not tell you. Consider this the solicited advice (presumably, if you are reading this chapter) that we have amassed from our combined years of trial and error as we each have pursued different paths in the field of forensic psychology.

Myth of the "Dream Job": Embracing the Glass Half Full

In an age where the Great Resignation (Parker & Horowitz, 2022) happened only a few years ago—and with one needing only to look so far as your social media feed for countless examples of people who have successfully created their "dream job" (and somehow done so by 21 years old?)—it can seem even more daunting to make a career choice. As with all things, picking a professional setting is a matter of compromise. Across our team of co-authors, we have yet to find a job role that includes all the aspects that we wanted to incorporate, at exactly the rate we wanted, and without any frustrating parts. In fact, we would wager that even those who have successfully built or obtained a "dream career" have their moments of frustration, failure, and frantic searches of www.indeed.com for open job positions on a particularly bad day. The grass is always greener, after all, and as psychologists, we know better than most that novelty wears off and humans habituate to even the most instrumental changes in life (Heshmat, 2014).

Instead of allowing yourself to get sucked into the myth of a "dream job," we encourage you to close out of your social media app or browser and take some time to identify the primary things *you* want your career to be about. If you could spend *most* of your time on any one responsibility, what would it be? Rather than focusing on finding the "perfect" career, focus on doing enough of what you love to offset the less romantic parts. Once you have found a setting that accommodates this, there are always ways to keep the remainder of your skillset alive and well (just read the next chapter of this book!). As will be discussed, in some settings, there may be room to negotiate stretch assignments (i.e., placements designed to develop skills outside of your current job description) or to protect time for additional projects or responsibilities, such as supervision or serving on a committee. It is also important to note that finding the right job is often an iterative process. You have different needs and goals at different points in your career. Perhaps your first job satisfies only a few of these (e.g., salary, location), but your second job can satisfy even more.

Even if your job does not allow for this type of negotiation, you can leverage hours outside the traditional work week if this is important to you. Can you spend time pursuing a passion project on the side? Maybe you want to write opinion pieces for a publication or work on a book proposal.

You might be wondering how you go about finding opportunities outside of your job. Maintaining relationships from your graduate program or training, continuing to network, and keeping a pulse on the field through involvement with organizations like the American Psychology-Law Society (AP-LS) are all routes to keeping the door open to opportunities. You can also leverage networking within your organization. This can open more routes than you might imagine, although it is often a waiting game. Volunteer your time and expertise to projects of interest, and they can turn into larger-scale opportunities or protected time to pursue a new route. In fact, every career opportunity this one co-author has had has directly resulted from taking advantage of an opportunity when it was offered as an add-on outside of the traditional work week. One thing that is important to keep in mind is that some jobs have non-compete clauses that prohibit you from working on certain projects or with certain organizations. Be sure to review your contract carefully when pursuing opportunities outside of your job.

Myth of Working Toward a Singular Outcome: Pursuing the Road Less Traveled

When your chosen career requires training as extensive and predetermined as that of a forensic psychologist, it can often feel—and, when you look around you, appear—as though there is one final career outcome. Indeed, for years, we all seem to be moving toward the same proverbial light at the end of the grueling graduate school tunnel. This is a limiting belief. The world is continuously changing and so is the workforce. Many of the authors of this book would not have envisioned a clinical career that could be primarily remote when we started our doctorate training, and yet . . . 2020 happened. Your career can take many forms over your lifetime, and it may not even follow one that you currently see modeled around you. Heck, it may not even be one that was covered in this book. But bear in mind that this sort of shape-shifting is not possible without intention, effort, hard work, perseverance, and often, risk and creativity.

Myth of Staying the (Ill-Suited) Course: Deciding When to Explore Other Options

Although a stable career in one organization is appealing to some, switching jobs is not the kiss of death it was once considered (Farmiloe, 2023). It is true that a resume with ten different jobs over a ten-year period may raise red flags to a potential employer, and recruiters appear to agree upon two years as a general rule for demonstrating dedication as an employee (Farmiloe, 2023). However, others note that, depending on the circumstance, staying in a job for two years just to put the time in may not always be advisable, particularly if you find yourself in a toxic work environment or in a role that is not consistent with your job description (Farmiloe, 2023). Just as your employer will not have a complete sense of you as a professional and individual from the interview process alone, there is only so much you can learn about your supervisor or organization prior to accepting a job. As noted, this is not a free pass to not do your due diligence but instead a reminder to be flexible and to not overestimate the gravity or permanence of a singular decision. Instead, we recommend explicitly expressing what you are interested in pursuing and asking about opportunities for this type of professional development during the interview stage. It can also be helpful to request to speak with different employees about their experience at the organization.

Ultimately, if a job is not working for you, is stagnating your professional development, or is overly stressful and/or toxic, there is no hard-and-fast rule about the number of years that you must remain with an organization before moving on. We certainly do not advise that you try careers on for size and leave in the amount of time it took you to apply for and accept the job. Making your career choices with intention is important, as is maintaining a good reputation and strong relationships with your colleagues and employers. However, it is also important to keep in mind that it is within your power to change your circumstances as needed.

Myth of Saying "Yes" to Everything: Leaning Into Intentional "Nos"

Many of us have been told that we should say "yes" to every opportunity that is presented to us to maximize our potential and grow as professionals. Although calling this a myth may seem to conflict with some of what we have discussed in this book—including the recommendation to seek opportunities to continue growing your skillset outside of your work hours—it is critical to remember that everything you say "yes" to is a "no" to something else. After all, we all have the same number of hours in the day, and everything you choose to do takes from elsewhere, whether professional or personal. It is a zero-sum process. It can be helpful to prioritize the job responsibilities that are most important to you and are achievable so that you can guide your decisions when taking on additional responsibilities. We will discuss more about approaches to supplemental opportunities and how to balance those opportunities in the next chapter.

If you take one thing away from our wisdom amassed across our joint years of trial and error, we hope it is this: remain flexible and open-minded as you embark on your career, and trust in the robust, comprehensive training that you have received. There is no one set of rules to follow to create a "perfect" career in one fell swoop. Our careers and our career goals evolve considerably over the course of our lifetimes. If you begin to challenge your limiting beliefs around your career—whether generated by yourself or others—you can begin to explore opportunities that may not have seemed within the realm of possibility.

YOUR CAREER PATH MAGIC WAND

Speaking of limiting beliefs, the last thing we leave you with in this chapter is a thought exercise intended to push you beyond the boundaries and barriers you may currently be facing. Borrowing from Acceptance and Commitment

Therapy (ACT; Hayes et al., 2016), we recommend using the magic wand exercise to envision your dream career as a forensic psychologist:

> Take a few minutes to imagine what your career would look like if you did not have any limits placed on you, even expanding beyond the advice and insight already provided in this book. In other words, what would your career look like if truly anything were possible?

Take this list and identify the "non-negotiables," the things you absolutely need in a job opportunity. This list can also include things that you absolutely cannot have in a job. This will help you concretely narrow down your options.

Next, identify the components that you want to continue to strive toward, either regardless of the setting or by finding ways to formally incorporate it into your work week. This list will keep moving you in the direction of your "dream career" even if no such Eden exists. It can also help you to decide among multiple seemingly equivalent job offers.

Continue to use this list as your North Star, or a grounding tool, to return to when you are in the thick of the stress of applications, interviews, and job negotiations. You can also revisit this throughout your career as a reminder of what you want for yourself while you are knee-deep in the responsibilities of your job or negotiating new opportunities for yourself.

CHAPTER TAKEAWAYS

Selecting the most appropriate career setting for you is deeply personal and nonetheless influenced by others around you (including the authors of books like this one). We hope that this chapter provided useful, practical insights, as well as prompts for self-reflection. Take time to prioritize both the professional *and* to prioritize the personal. Make sure you engage in myth busting and do not blindly accept what appear to be career constraints. And remember, there is always room to grow and transform your career as long as you approach decision making intentionally.

REFERENCES

Farmiloe, B. (2023, July 5). How long should you stay at a job? *Fast Company.* https://www.fastcompany.com/90917028/how-long-should-you-stay-at-a-job

Federal Student Aid. (n.d.). *Public Service Loan Forgiveness (PSLF).* https://studentaid.gov/manage-loans/forgiveness-cancellation/public-service

Goff-Dupont, S. (2022, January 12). The truth about compressed workweeks, according to people who've done it. *Atlassian.* https://www.atlassian.com/blog/productivity/compressed-work-week-how-to

Hatcher, R. L., Wise, E. H., & Grus, C. L. (2015). Preparation for practicum in professional psychology: A survey of training directors. *Training and Education in Professional Psychology*, *9*(1), 5–12. https://doi.org/10.1037/tep0000060

Hayes, S. C., Strosahl, K. D., & Wilson, K. G. (2016). *Acceptance and commitment therapy: The process and practice of mindful change* (2nd ed.). The Guilford Press.

Heshmat, S. (2014, December 30). Change and habituation: On taking things for granted. *Psychology Today*. https://www.psychologytoday.com/us/blog/science-choice/201412/change-and-habituation

Parker, K., & Horowitz, J. M. (2022, March 9). Majority of workers who quit a job in 2021 cite low pay, no opportunities for advancement, feeling disrespected. *Pew Research Center*. https://www.pewresearch.org/short-reads/2022/03/09/majority-of-workers-who-quit-a-job-in-2021-cite-low-pay-no-opportunities-for-advancement-feeling-disrespected/

Parker, K., Horowitz, J. M., & Minkin, R. (2022, February 16). COVID-19 pandemic continues to reshape work in America. *Pew Research Center*. https://www.pewresearch.org/social-trends/2022/02/16/covid-19-pandemic-continues-to-reshape-work-in-america/

Ramsey, M. (2023, September 15). Emerging trends in paid leave offer new support for employees. *The Society for Human Resources Management*. https://www.shrm.org/topics-tools/news/all-things-work/expanding-view-paid-leave

VA Careers. (n.d.). *Education support*. https://vacareers.va.gov/employment-benefits/education-support/

CHAPTER 11

I Want to Do Everything! Creating/Pursuing Supplemental Opportunities to Round Out Your Career and Life Experience

Thus far, the major focus of this book has been providing readers with the information needed to select the best *home base* for their career in forensic psychology. Given that work occupies roughly half of our waking hours on most days, the decision as to where one's career home base will be is a massive one. That said, it is rare that selecting the most appropriate home base for yourself means that *all* your professional itches are scratched. In other words, very few jobs are the vaunted "perfect fit" that check off all the boxes regarding your interests and passions in forensic psychology. Rather, the choice of the most appropriate home base tends to encompass a job that checks most of your boxes (or at least checks off the most important boxes).

Surely, this must mean you are doomed to a career and life that is not completely in balance with your interests and passions, right? Not to fret—with some creativity, there are plenty of ways to make sure that you are able to achieve fulfillment in the areas of forensic psychology that are important to you. This chapter focuses on highlighting side opportunities in forensic psychology that are lower-burden and have relatively few barriers to entry. Specifically, it will explore these opportunities in three domains: (1) scholarship, (2) teaching and mentoring, and (3) clinical work. Hopefully, when you are done reading this chapter, you will be able to brainstorm the career path that makes the most sense for you, both in terms of your home base *and* in terms of the supplemental professional opportunities you choose to pursue.

DOI: 10.4324/9781003408857-16

SUPPLEMENTAL OPPORTUNITIES IN SCHOLARSHIP

As explored earlier in this book (Chapters 4 and 5), regular contribution to scholarship is most commonly a job expectation in academic settings. But what if you are not an academic where part of your job time is expected to be contributing to forensic psychology's literature base? Are you unable to express your love of scholarship if you do not have the time to pursue grants, conduct research studies, or serve as a lead author on peer-reviewed articles? By now, you should be noticing a common theme across this book; there are *multiple paths* to a fulfilling professional life, and those paths are easier to maximize with some *creativity*. If you are a professional who does not have allotted job time to contribute to scholarship, later are some suggested pathways as to how you might be able to still contribute to scholarship in forensic psychology without destroying your work-life balance.

Contributing Authorship

The gold standard contribution to the literature base in forensic psychology is the peer-reviewed publication. Reflecting that they are the gold standard, these are perhaps the most difficult types of publications to get. They require submission to only one journal at a time. Each submission typically requires a lengthy review and revision process. Additionally, for many journals—particularly those with higher impact factors—acceptance rates are low, meaning that it often takes multiple attempts to get a manuscript published. Further still, once a manuscript is accepted, there are several rounds of proofing that need to be completed to make it ready for prime time.

The aforementioned seemingly makes achieving publication of a peer-reviewed article look like a burdensome process that can constitute a major time commitment. That is true—*at least for the lead author*. Generally, the submission, revision, and proofing process for a peer-reviewed publication has one point person—usually, the lead (or corresponding) author. In contrast, contributing authors typically help with some aspect of writing the manuscript but are not responsible for the remainder of the process (save contributing to requested revisions). In short, contributing authors help with only the primary task of writing, not the secondary task of going through the rigmarole of publication procedure (though there are exceptions, such as when a contributing author is a student and assists the lead author with secondary tasks in order to gain valuable experience). As such, serving as a contributing author is usually less time-intensive than serving as a lead author, and it is something that is easier to integrate into your schedule in a way that can maintain work-life balance. The upside? You can contribute to the gold standard of scholarship in forensic psychology. The downside? You may not get the same name recognition as the lead author. If you enjoy working on peer-reviewed scholarship—but you do not have room in your schedule for the duties of a lead author and do not place great value in name recognition—looking for opportunities to be a contributing author might be a great strategy for you.

Non-Peer-Reviewed Publications

You do not have to do things to the "gold standard" to make valuable contributions to a profession. The very term "gold standard" invokes thoughts of precious metals, with gold being at the top of the hierarchy. But ask yourself this: If someone came to you and offered you either bronze or silver, would you really turn it down *just* because they did not offer you gold? Alternatively, do you view it as a magnificent accomplishment to win an Olympic bronze or silver metal? If you answered "no" to the first question and/or "yes" to the second question, you might consider pursuing publications that are not subject to an intensive peer review process. Here, we will explore three types of publications that are not subject to a lengthy peer review process: (1) book chapters, (2) industry magazine articles, and (3) industry newsletter articles.

After peer-reviewed publications, books and book chapters are likely the next most respected types of scholarship to which a forensic psychologist can contribute. Books and book chapters often focus on one of two things: (1) summarizing a research base regarding a forensic psychology topic or (2) highlighting practical applications of forensic psychology concepts. Given that this chapter reviews opportunities to *supplement* your "9 to 5" to achieve professional wholeness, time commitment is a key concern. For that reason, it is not suggested that writing a full book is a good supplemental opportunity. A book chapter, on the other hand, just might be.

A benefit of writing book chapters is that *novel* contributions to scholarship are not an expectation (though they may happen). Rather, as stated earlier, book chapters often call for summarizing a literature base or discussing how a concept applies in certain settings. Book chapters do not require having applied for a grant and conducting a research study. Further, although they may require a revision process, it is substantially less intensive than that of a peer-reviewed article. Further still, book chapters are typically not blind submissions that are subject to a gatekeeping process. Rather, book chapters are typically invited or solicited and, except in rare cases, are guaranteed publication.

In the former case (invited), an editor of a book may reach out to you with a chapter topic because they are familiar with your expertise in a certain area. A common example is that of a handbook, where an editor has a clear topic/theme in mind. The editors invite authors who they think can do justice to a topic they want to include in the handbook. An example is *Learning Forensic Assessment: Research and Practice* (2nd ed.) (Jackson & Roesch, 2016), a handbook published in Routledge's *International Perspectives on Forensic Mental Health Series*. In the latter case (solicited), editors may put out a call (often, via a progressional group's listserv or newsletter) asking for authors to submit ideas for a chapter. This is more common in a volume-based series, where topics covered in the book do not necessarily have to relate to each other. In forensic psychology, an example of this type of book is the *Advances in Psychology & Law* series published by Springer.

Still seem like too much? You could always pair a book chapter with the strategy discussed directly earlier and be a contributing author. Generally, this requires you to write a portion of the chapter and to provide feedback on the work of other authors, but it absolves you of the responsibility of coordinating and editing contributions of co-authors and of navigating the submission and proofing process (which, even though less burdensome, can still require substantial time commitment).

Two other good options to contribute to scholarship beyond peer-reviewed articles and book chapters are publishing in *industry magazines* or *industry newsletters*. As with book chapters, publication in these media generally does not require novel contributions to scholarship in the field. In contrast to book chapters, though, industry magazine and newsletter articles are typically significantly shorter and less comprehensive. Often, the writing burden reflects hours and days, not weeks and months. Additionally, like book chapters, such articles are generally either invited or solicited and reflect publications that are virtually guaranteed. A detriment to writing for these forums is that it does not command the same type of prestige or recognition as publishing a peer-reviewed article or a book chapter, as the publication process is less rigorous. However, an oft-overlooked benefit of these types of media is *reach*.

Accessibility has become a popular topic in forensic psychology. Just as it can be difficult for individuals with mental health challenges and justice involvement to access high-quality forensic psychology services, it can also be difficult for professionals to access the forensic psychology literature base. If one is not an academic, access to peer-reviewed journal articles can require expensive subscriptions to research databases. Additionally, access to book chapters generally requires the purchasing of a book in whole or in part. Some books come with hefty price tags (i.e., hundreds of dollars), particularly in hardcover format. In contrast, industry magazine and newsletter articles are often substantially easier to access. Their access may be a perk that is included with membership to a professional organization (e.g., a state or regional psychological association, the American Psychological Association). Better still, access may be free, even to individuals who are not members of a professional organization. A salient example of this is the *American Psychology-Law Society Newsletter*, which is published free of charge on AP-LS's website (www.ap-ls.org/newsletter). As the accessibility of these media is greater and readership may be higher, authors of magazine and newsletter articles may have greater reach than authors of book chapters or peer-reviewed articles. For those who are not overly concerned with recognition and who have more limited time to contribute to scholarship, seeking to publish in an industry magazine or newsletter may be a solid option.

EXAMPLES OF FORENSIC MENTAL HEALTH MAGAZINES AND NEWSLETTERS

- *American Psychology-Law Society Newsletter* (APA Div. 41)
- *Forward* (APA Div. 9)
- *International Association for Correctional and Forensic Psychology Bulletin*
- *International Association of Forensic Mental Health Services Newsletter*
- *The Gavel* (APA Div. 18)
- *Monitor on Psychology Judicial Notebook Column* (APA Div. 9)

Research and Professional Conferences

Writing is not the only method for disseminating scholarly work. If you are someone who enjoys presenting more than writing, submitting your work to research and professional conferences can be a great way to contribute to scholarship. Generally, submission to conferences is refereed, meaning that you submit an idea and are not guaranteed a presentation spot. However, the submission is typically in the form of an abstract, which is a short summary of your proposed work and a much less intensive writing burden than if submitting a piece for publication. Acceptance of a proposal requires preparing a presentation (a talk or a poster). Though this requires time, it is generally less time-consuming than authoring a peer-reviewed publication or a book chapter. As a benefit, conferences are a great forum for professional networking; presenting at a conference can help you stand out. As another added benefit, conferences are often held in interesting locations. If you like presenting and you have an itch to travel, submitting to and presenting at research and professional conferences might be a great way to quench both thirsts.

EXAMPLES OF FORENSIC MENTAL HEALTH MAGAZINES AND NEWSLETTERS

- *American Psychology-Law Society Newsletter* (APA Div. 41)
- *Forward* (APA Div. 9)
- *International Association for Correctional and Forensic Psychology Bulletin*
- *International Association of Forensic Mental Health Services Newsletter*
- *The Gavel* (APA Div. 18)
- *Monitor on Psychology Judicial Notebook Column* (APA Div. 9)

Reviewing for Journals

Feel like you do not have time to write or present anything? Believe it or not, you can still contribute to scholarship. This can be accomplished by serving as a peer reviewer. Serving as a peer reviewer allows an individual to review manuscripts that are within their area of expertise. It allows an individual to contribute to psychology's gatekeeping function while also allowing individuals to provide valuable feedback to authors that can help them improve the rigor of their work and its impact on the field. Additionally, the time commitment for serving as a peer reviewer—provided you do not have designs on becoming a member of an editorial board or becoming an associate editor—is generally only an hour or two at a time.

EXAMPLE JOURNALS FORENSIC PSYCHOLOGISTS MIGHT REVIEW FOR

- *Behavioral Sciences & the Law*
- *Criminal Behaviour and Mental Health*
- *Criminal Justice and Behavior*
- *Forensic and Legal Psychology*
- *International Journal of Forensic Mental Health*
- *Journal of Forensic Psychology: Research and Practice*
- *Law and Human Behavior*
- *Legal and Criminological Psychology*

SUPPLEMENTAL OPPORTUNITIES IN TEACHING AND MENTORSHIP

As with publishing, teaching and mentoring is an expected job duty predominantly in academic settings (see Chapters 4 and 5). However, that does not mean that other settings cannot offer opportunities to teach and mentor! For example, it is not uncommon for clinical settings—particularly group private practices or public sector clinical sites—to offer training programs like pre-doctoral internships and postdoctoral fellowships. These can offer great opportunities for individuals to supervise and mentor trainees in clinical work, contribute to the training program's didactic series, or supervise and mentor trainees in scholarly work. To this end, the Student Committee of the American Psychology-Law Society maintains and regularly updates databases of various pre-doctoral internship and postdoctoral fellowship programs in forensic psychology (see http://www.apls-students.org/). For individuals interested predominantly in clinical work—but who would like for part of their career experience to be teaching and mentoring trainees—targeting employment at one of these sites is a sound strategy.

The earlier example demonstrates how one might pursue supplemental opportunities *within* one's home base. However, the focus of this chapter is mainly on pursuing supplemental opportunities if your home base does not provide such opportunities. Thankfully, supplemental opportunities to teach and mentor in forensic psychology are abundant. We will review three possibilities here: (1) serving as an adjunct professor, (2) serving as a volunteer faculty member, and (3) pursuing one-off teaching opportunities.

Adjunct Professor

If you love teaching classes—but your home base is not in academia—a supplemental opportunity of interest to you might be that of an adjunct professor (also known as contingent faculty or adjunct lecturer). Adjunct professors are part-time employees who typically teach only one course at a time at an institution (as opposed to juggling multiple classes). These positions are common, representing 44% of all faculty positions at postsecondary institutions (National Center for Education Statistics, 2023), and they exist at nearly every institution. Although they lack some benefits associated with full-fledged professors, such as health insurance and job security, adjunct faculty positions can offer notable advantages. First, adjunct faculty have minimal obligations beyond their courses. Attendance at faculty meetings, committee service, and academic advising are often optional. Second, adjunct positions provide significant flexibility. Adjunct professors can choose where and which courses to teach and have greater flexibility in selecting times they would like to teach. Some may teach at multiple institutions; some may even opt to teach only virtually (Goldman & Schmalz, 2012). For those enthusiastic about teaching but who have no interest in being a full-time professor, an adjunct position may be ideal.

Volunteer Faculty

Another method of affiliating with a university—but that typically does not require formally teaching classes—is that of a volunteer faculty appointment (also commonly referred to as a "courtesy appointment," "visiting faculty member," or "clinical faculty," depending on the setting). Volunteer faculty are those whose affiliation is recognized by an academic department, but they are not compensated faculty. Rather, they volunteer their time to the department. To qualify for volunteer faculty appointments, individuals generally must make substantial contributions to the department and to the student experience. Examples of substantial contributions include collaboration on scholarship, serving on thesis and dissertation committees, conducting didactic lectures, or supervising clinical rotations. These types of appointments generally require nomination by a salaried faculty member in the department and wider department (and often dean) approval. Benefits of being a volunteer faculty vary across institutions. For some institutions, ability to list them as an academic affiliation is the main benefit. For others, volunteer faculty may qualify for an institutional email address and be granted access to research databases. Regardless, if you are interested in an academic affiliation—but do not necessarily want to consistently teach courses—pursuing a volunteer faculty appointment may represent a good option.

Guest Lectures, Didactics, and Continuing Education

A third pathway to integrating teaching and mentorship into your professional career if it is not an established expectation at your job is to devote time to one-off teaching opportunities. As has been a theme throughout this chapter, a major benefit of providing one-off teaching is that it is a relatively low time commitment. Typically, the time commitment reflects the length of the presentation and the preparation time for the presentation; this is usually only a few hours. Those who really enjoy teaching can look for these opportunities with greater frequency, which encompasses a greater time commitment. However, it is easy to engage in this type of teaching infrequently but consistently (e.g., one or two times per year). For many, this may be enough to scratch the teaching itch without proving overly burdensome to work-life balance.

Many and varied opportunities exist to provide one-off teaching. Common examples might include providing a guest lecture for a forensic psychology course, providing a didactic lecture for a clinical training program (such as a pre-doctoral internship, a postdoctoral fellowship program, or a psychiatry residency program), or providing a continuing education didactic for a state or regional professional association. The last option may provide opportunities for cross-disciplinary teaching, as many professions benefit from didactic lectures on psycholegal topics (e.g., social work, counseling, psychiatry).

One type of one-off teaching activity that bears special mention is that of providing continuing legal education (CLEs) or continuing judicial education (CJEs). Like psychologists, attorneys and judges have an obligation to stay current in their field and must complete a certain number of CLEs/CJEs over specified periods of time. CLEs/CJEs are a great way to develop skills at translating complex psychological topics for non-mental health audiences. In other words, CLEs/CJEs can be very helpful in developing the *translational skillset* that can be very useful for forensic psychologists who are often interfacing with legal professionals (particularly psychologists who testify in court regularly). In addition to helping forensic psychologists develop translational skillsets, volunteering your time for CLEs/CJEs is also a great *marketing tool*. Teaching CLEs/CJEs exposes you to individuals who may send you referrals. CLEs/CJEs allow you to showcase your expertise as a forensic psychologist. They also allow legal professionals to get a sense of how you are as a public speaker, which is particularly important when attorneys and courts are looking for experts who they think will deliver both good written work and good testimony. If you are interested in providing CLEs/CJEs, reaching out to local public defender offices, local prosecutor offices, local or state bar associations, local law practices, or local or state judges associations may be good possibilities.

SUPPLEMENTAL OPPORTUNITIES IN CLINICAL WORK

Earlier, we reviewed supplemental opportunities regarding scholarship and regarding teaching/mentoring. Truthfully, these types of supplemental opportunities are both more plentiful and are easier to manage in terms of work-life balance. In contrast, supplemental opportunities in clinical work often tend to be more time-consuming and less plentiful. They may require more effort on your part in terms of finding opportunities. That said, these opportunities do exist. We will explore three here: (1) side private practice, (2) part-time clinical employment, and (3) pro bono practice.

Side Private Practice

We reviewed private practice as a career home base in Chapter 7. Having a side private practice just means having a part-time private practice. As such, similar concerns apply regarding full-time private practice as side private practice in terms of generating referrals, managing a business, etc. However, having a side private practice means that you have a career home base that is *not* a private practice. Most likely, then, you have a steady income that you are looking to supplement with your side practice. That takes off substantial pressure, as the side practice is not your main source of income. In essence, you have greater "wiggle room" so to speak with a side practice as you will not be wholly dependent upon that income to support yourself. This may allow you to be more selective with the clinical work you pursue, as well as provide you with greater flexibility as to when you choose to pursue it. Common examples of side practices are academics who maintain a part-time private practice, a public sector psychologist who negotiates a compressed schedule to allow time to conduct forensic mental health assessments on the side, or individuals with traditional work schedules and who provide therapy services several evenings per week.

Part-Time Clinical Employment

Part-time clinical employment refers to maintaining a clinical job as your second job. Given that your part-time clinical practice is a form of employment, the hours allotted are usually more consistent and structured than if you were to maintain a side private practice. As examples, such opportunities may include working a compressed schedule for your primary job on Monday through Thursday but then completing forensic assessments on Fridays at a state hospital, on a psychiatric ward in a community hospital, or for a court clinic. A benefit of part-time clinical employment is that it generates extra money and may be easier in terms of life planning (in that hours and income are more consistent). A downside, however, is that it may be less flexible than maintaining a side private practice. In other words, you may not have the same flexibility to forego clinical work to do other things (such as taking a long weekend for leisure travel).

Pro Bono Practice

A final supplemental opportunity for clinical work is pro bono practice. Pro bono practice can best be thought of as utilizing your forensic psychology background for charitable/service purposes. In fact, the *Specialty Guidelines for Forensic Psychology* emphasize pro bono service, with Guideline 5.03 reading, "Forensic psychologists recognize that some persons may have limited access to legal services as a function of financial disadvantage and strive to contribute a portion of their professional time for little or no compensation or personal advantage" (American Psychological Association, 2013). Although pro bono is often equated with providing free services, providing low-cost services (sometimes called "low bono") is also often recognized as pro bono service.

A context in which pro bono forensic mental health assessments are more common is immigration, particularly asylum. Individuals seek to immigrate into the United States for a multitude of reasons. Unfortunately, those reasons sometimes involve seeking refuge from traumatic circumstances. An in-depth discussion of forensic mental health assessment in immigration contexts is beyond the scope of this book, other than to reference that pro bono service is more common in this context. For a comprehensive review of how forensic psychologists may provide services in immigration contexts, we recommend exploring the work of Barber-Rioja et al. (2022) and Evans and Hass (2018).

Though we will not be providing an overview of evaluations in immigration contexts, we are happy to provide some leads as to how forensic psychologists may get involved in such evaluations. Several organizations host networks of psychologists, physicians, and other mental health professionals who provide pro bono evaluations to asylum seekers. Salient examples include the Mount Sinai Human Rights Program (www.mountsinaihumanrights.org), where forensic psychologists can provide virtual evaluations to asylum seekers, as well as Physicians for Human Rights (www.phr.org), where forensic psychologists provide in-person evaluations after being contacted by a local asylum attorney. Not familiar with asylum evaluations? Not to worry—both organizations provide training for all volunteer evaluators!

EXAMPLES OF OTHER ORGANIZATIONS THAT PROVIDE PRO BONO ASYLUM EVALUATIONS

- Columbia Human Rights Initiatives Asylum Clinic (New York, NY)
- Evaluation Alliance for Human Rights (AZ and WA)
- HEAL Refugee Health & Asylum Collaborative (Baltimore, MD)
- New Mexico Immigrant Law Center (Albuquerque, NM)
- Philadelphia Human Rights Clinic (Philadelphia, PA)

CHAPTER TAKEAWAYS

Choosing the most appropriate "home base" for your career in forensic mental health is challenging. Rarely will your career home base fulfill *all* your professional, interests, desires, and aspirations. However, with some creativity, you can pursue supplemental opportunities that will help you to actualize as a forensic psychologist. For those seeking supplemental scholarship opportunities, serving as a contributing author, pursuing non-peer-reviewed publications, presenting at research and professional conferences, and serving as a peer reviewer for academic journals in forensic psychology are solid options. For those seeking supplemental teaching and mentoring opportunities, serving as an adjunct professor, serving as a volunteer faculty member, or pursuing one-off teaching opportunities (e.g., didactic trainings, continuing education trainings) in forensic psychology may prove fruitful. Finally, for those seeking supplemental clinical opportunities, maintaining a side private practice, having a part-time clinical job, or completing pro bono evaluations (such as for asylum seekers) may be viable strategies.

REFERENCES

American Psychological Association. (2013). Specialty guidelines for forensic psychology. *American Psychologist, 68*(1), 7–19. https://doi.org/10.1037/a0029889

Barber-Rioja, V., Akinsulure-Smith, A. M., & Vendzules, S. (2022). *Mental health evaluations in immigration courts: A guide for mental health and legal professionals.* NYU Press.

Evans, F. B., & Hass, G. A. (2018). *Forensic psychological assessment in immigration court: A guidebook for evidence-based and ethical practice.* Routledge. https://doi.org/10.4324/9781315621197

Goldman, K. D., & Schmalz, K. J. (2012). Adjunct teaching: Part-time professorial possibilities, provisions, and provisos. *Health Promotion Practice, 13*(3), 301–307. https://doi.org/10.1177/1524839912442516

Jackson, R., & Roesch, R. (Eds.). (2016). *Learning forensic assessment: Research and Practice* (2nd ed.). Routledge.

National Center for Education Statistics. (2023). *Characteristics of postsecondary faculty.* https://nces.ed.gov/programs/coe/indicator/csc/postsecondary-faculty

CHAPTER 12

Representing Forensic Psychology Regardless of Setting

Do's & Don'ts for a Successful Career

We hope that *Career Paths in Forensic Psychology* has provided you with insights and tips that broaden your horizons and enable you to thrive in your forensic psychology career of choice. With this added knowledge, you may have clarity into your ideal job activities and settings, or you may benefit from additional time to mull over your options. However, regardless of what form your career as a forensic psychologist assumes, one thing will hold true: maintaining a strong professional reputation is of the utmost importance.

Who we are as professionals reflects not only on our mentors and institutions but also on the field of forensic psychology as a whole. Individuals' experiences with forensic psychologists can influence their belief in the need to address mental health in the legal system and their trust in this field, which may be more salient than ever given the focus in recent years on "true crime" and misconduct in the criminal justice system. Further, the subfield of forensic psychology is in its early stages relative to the broader field of psychology. This world often is a small one. Professional and personal networks are extensive, people talk, and your reputation very well may follow you throughout your career.

With this in mind, we thought it prudent to leave you with recommendations on representing the field of forensic psychology, putting your best foot forward as a professional, and ensuring your success over time. In this final chapter, we will discuss ethical and best practices for forensic psychology, as well as factors related to overall professionalism and career satisfaction over time.

DOI: 10.4324/9781003408857-17

PRACTICE GUIDELINES: ETHICAL AND BEST PRACTICES FOR FORENSIC PSYCHOLOGY

Our training as psychologists inherently shapes the ethical lens we apply across our careers, regardless of work environment. At minimum, if you are working in a clinical capacity, you should always be aware of the laws governing the state in which you are practicing (see DeMatteo et al., in press). However, beyond state and federal laws, psychologists have codes of ethics and conduct that inform our actions as professionals and, in some cases, can serve as the basis for sanctions if violated. For example, members of the American Psychological Association are expected to adhere to the standards set forth in the *Ethical Principles of Psychologists and Code of Conduct* (referred to as the Ethics Code). Other entities, such as state psychological associations or licensing boards, may sanction psychologists who are found to have violated Ethics Code standards (APA, 2017). Further, most states have adopted the Ethics Code into law governing psychological practice.

Reviewing professional standards and guidelines in detail is beyond the scope of this book, but we recommend familiarizing (or refamiliarizing—refreshers are never a bad thing!) yourself with both the APA *Ethical Principles of Psychologists and Code of Conduct* and the more specific *Specialty Guidelines for Forensic Psychology* (referred to as the Specialty Guidelines). However, we wanted to highlight a few central tenets to illustrate the types of considerations that should be front of mind for psychologists across professional settings.

A NOTE ON STANDARDS VERSUS PRINCIPLES

The APA Ethics Code is organized into standards and principles. Knowing the distinction between them is paramount to protecting yourself from liability as a psychologist. Standards are mandatory practices that may be enforceable by law, whereas principles are aspirational recommendations for how to promote best practices. Thus, standards are necessary to follow, and principles are something to strive toward.

Psychologists are guided by the principles of beneficence (i.e., promoting good) and nonmaleficence (i.e., avoiding harm), fidelity and responsibility, integrity, justice, and respect for people's rights and dignity (APA, 2017). Forensic psychologists must also bear in mind the added responsibilities inherent to our nuanced role within the legal system. When working with justice-involved individuals, the ripple effects of our professional choices and practices can be huge!

Enter the Specialty Guidelines, which highlight the importance of attending to conflicts of interest, impartiality, pressure, and bias within the forensic realm: "Forensic practitioners strive for accuracy, honesty, and truthfulness in the science, teaching and practice of forensic psychology and they strive to resist partisan pressures to provide services in any ways that might tend to be misleading or accurate" (APA, 2013, p. 8). As highlighted in the Specialty Guidelines, although we often view these practices as important for more traditional psychology roles (e.g., clinician), these considerations can arise across settings and may not always be in line with the organization in which you are working. As psychologists, we have a responsibility to center these considerations across professional roles when practicing our trade, even if we do not have the word "psychologist" in our title.

It might come as a surprise to you that our Ethics Codes and Specialty Guidelines can present a source of conflict depending on your work setting. After all, these concepts seem quite straightforward at face value. Don't we all strive to achieve accuracy and honesty? Aren't we all aiming to do right by our work and the communities or clients we serve? Conflicts may be more common than you would think, particularly in the absence of the structured spaces for group supervision, consultation, and classroom discussion that we are used to. So how might living out these principles look in practice? What's it really like out there?

With more and more psychologists leaving academia and healthcare for the corporate world (Novotney, 2022), some of us may find ourselves in environments where objectivity and data-driven decision making are not the norm. Instead, profit, timelines, deliverables, and pre-established measures of success may dictate an organization's efforts. For example, many organizations have begun to incorporate in-house research, and user-focused (UX) research has become an increasingly common lucrative career option. However, the training, function, and goals behind this kind of research do not necessarily align with that of scientists and doctorate-level researchers. So if you find yourself in an UX research role, you may struggle to rectify a preference for comprehensive research practices versus research practices with more convenient methodologies and quicker turnaround times. Taking this a step further, our professional standards direct our interpretation and representation of research findings, which may create conflict in situations where the research does not necessarily reflect what a company had in mind when embarking on a project.

Another example concerns the client, consumer, or community on which your work focuses. If you were tasked with conducting an internal research project or promoting staff well-being, the standards of beneficence and non-maleficence may lead you to make recommendations that are consistent with psychologists' best practices but in conflict with what your boss or company wants to hear. For example, is the company taking care not to publish names alongside customer feedback if the survey was presented as anonymous? Are surveys within the organization being designed with validity and reliability in mind? Are we asking the right questions to inform the insights the organization is claiming to obtain versus the ones it hopes to receive? These are all the types of questions that you may find yourself faced with in professional settings, where doctorate-level psychologists and researchers are not the norm. If these examples leave you deeply concerned about the state of the corporate world, it is important to remember that our training was niche and specialized, with the highest practice standards and ethics in mind. We cannot simply expect others to have this same understanding, even if they want to do everything right. Instead, we should consider ways to raise these considerations, disseminate this knowledge, and advocate for best practices.

"SOFT SKILLS" IN THE WORKPLACE: ACHIEVING SUCCESS THROUGH INTERPERSONAL SKILLS

You may be feeling a bit dejected. After all, we dropped two hard truths about life as a forensic psychologist: (1) Even if you want to transition fully to a non-traditional workplace, if your work is still forensic in nature (e.g., focused on mental health policy, working with justice-involved communities), you are still a forensic psychologist, and (2) not everyone is going to view things the same way as our field does.

Accepting that this very well may be your experience at some point in your career, you may be wondering how to even go about best representing the field and navigating potential conflicts along the way. Don't worry—we've got you covered. (After all, we haven't let you down yet, have we?) This time, these recommendations come in the form of "soft skills," or the interpersonal skills that set us up for success in the workplace. When you find yourself caught in the inevitable workplace conflict, remember to rely on a few core skills: adaptability, communication, conflict resolution, and negotiation.

Adaptability

Adaptability is chief among the skills that will allow you to navigate challenging work situations and stressors with grace. Fortunately, this is a skill for which our pre- and postdoctoral training sets us up nicely, whether in the form of learning to pivot based on unexpected research findings, adjusting to the high-stress and often unpredictable nature of clinical care, or simply keeping up to date with the latest evidence base that informs our practice. If you can maintain a sense of psychological flexibility and readily adapt to changes in the workplace, you will be better off in navigating curveballs in the workplace.

Communication

In addition to the internal skills we can apply to help us through tough times at work, communication is key. In fact, a lot of conflict can arise from a lack of communication or transparency as people rush in to fill gaps in messaging, often with the worst-case scenario. Being clear and concise when collaborating with others is a useful skill and one that you cannot always take for granted. *Forbes* outlines a number of effective communication skills in the workplace, including active listening; embracing feedback; being clear, courteous, and open-minded in communication; and expressing gratitude (Jolaoso & Main, 2023).

Conflict Resolution

So what if you've done all the adapting you can and you communicated openly and respectfully, but you still find yourself embroiled in a workplace conflict? This is absolutely to be expected at some point in your career. After all, lots of personalities, life circumstances, motivations, personal and professional stressors, and needs collide in a workplace environment. Frankly, it's shocking that conflicts don't arise more frequently. It can be helpful to shift from a perspective of trying to avoid workplace conflict altogether (how exhausting!) and instead focus on how you resolve it when it does happen.

Oore and colleagues' (2015) review of successful conflict resolution reveals a range of helpful traits and perspectives. Fortunately, the clinical part of your training as a psychologist may actually have primed you to succeed in these areas, including cognitive flexibility, a balanced focus on self versus others, and emotion regulation (Oore et al., 2015). Sounds a lot like our third-wave behavioral therapies, doesn't it?

Negotiation

Once you've tapped into your clinical training to practice skills for internal regulation, there remains the matter of the other person, team, or topic at hand. As appealing as it can be to simply avoid the situation and solely manage our own reactions, it can be important to address the issue head on. Based on the issue and your goals, conflict resolution may consist of accommodating, compromising, or collaborating (Cote, 2023).

According to Cote (2023), accommodation is recommended when either your relationship with your colleague or de-escalating the situation is most important; however, the downsides to this approach are that it may involve you placing your ideas or workplace goals aside in an effort to avoid interpersonal difficulty. This can be the death of innovation, creativity, and collaboration in the workplace. Compromise, instead, involves both members conceding part of their goal so that a balance can be struck; this approach can be a useful way to meet both career and relationship goals simultaneously, although it is unlikely that you will be fully satisfied in either realm (Cote, 2023). Lastly, collaboration involves working together to find an outcome—likely one that has not already been discussed and hopefully one that can meet both needs in a satisfactory manner that is both professionally and personally fulfilling (Cote, 2023). Once again, these sound a lot like dialectical behavior therapy's DEAR MAN (describe, express, assert, reinforce, mindful, appear, negotiate; Linehan, 2015) interpersonal effectiveness skills. Life mirroring art.

THE BIGGER PICTURE: JOB SATISFACTION AND BURNOUT

You can carry yourself in the best ways you know how, with the integrity and responsibility emphasized in the Ethics Code and Specialty Guidelines and with interpersonal skills that serve you well across stressful work experiences. But as much as it pains us to say this, it's important to note that even with the best of efforts, we do not always land in a work environment that is a good fit, and there are many larger life contexts that can influence our experience in the workplace. Job dissatisfaction and burnout are possibilities worth keeping an eye out for.

The job market seems to increasingly be driven by expectations for promotion, pay increases, growth, and work-life balance. Job satisfaction may be more important than ever, and the absence of it has sparked trends, such as the Great Resignation (Parker & Horowitz, 2022), followed by less extreme, but nonetheless harmful, trends like "quiet quitting," "bare minimum Mondays," "resenteeism," and "rage applying" (Jackson, 2023). In case you find yourself wondering why nobody seems to want to work hard anymore, it's important to note that these trends don't occur in a vacuum and instead may in part reflect employer behaviors. Indeed, employers have similarly begun engaging in "quiet firing" and "quiet hiring." These practices are efforts to avoid having to provide resources, like severance pay, by making work requirements so undesirable that people eventually leave of their own accord or to avoid having to hire in bad economies by providing current employees with additional, uncompensated responsibilities (Jackson, 2023).

So for those of us who may find ourselves phoning it into our day jobs, adaptation, negotiation, and conflict resolution at all costs are not always the answer—particularly if making it work in your current job is no longer in your best interest personally or professionally. However, this doesn't necessarily mean you have no choice but to throw in the towel. There are ways to advocate for your own interests and needs in the workplace (or to make the decision to separate responsibly) while still maintaining good working relationships and demonstrating strong professionalism.

You may be comforted to know that, in contrast to these trends, practicing psychologists have largely reported job satisfaction across the years (e.g., Rupert et al., 2012), with primary predictors being earning potential (i.e., direct-pay clients), work-life balance, having a sense of control and agency, and having satisfying work experiences. Among VA Medical Centers, a sample of psychologists reported being somewhat satisfied on average and expressed low intent to leave (Yanchus et al., 2015). Respect, procedural justice, autonomy, and psychological safety were predictors of lower rates of turnover via their impact on job satisfaction (Yanchus et al., 2015).

How do these trends differ for forensic psychologists specifically? Forensic psychologists work with some of the most complex populations and in particularly challenging environments, like jails and prisons. Despite the popularity of and craze around true crime, the reality of working in the justice system and directly with affected populations is much more impactful and emotionally draining than listening to a podcast or watching a Netflix docuseries from the comfort of your home. There is no pause button or commercial break, and the realities of these life circumstances are often more complex and heartbreaking than what we are shown in popular media. These experiences take a very real toll. At the same time, we don't simply fall into these roles, but rather, we pursue them with tenacity and perseverance. Surely, after such intentional effort to become a forensic psychologist, we would land in a fulfilling and satisfying environment, right?

One study examined the experiences of 49 U.S. forensic psychologists who were sampled from the Society for Police and Criminal Psychology (SPCP), the American Academy of Forensic Sciences (AAFS), and APA Divisions 18, 39, 41, and 42 (Washington, 2019). This sample reported moderate-to-high levels of job satisfaction due to factors including the ability to keep busy, have independent work, enjoy diversity in their roles, live into values of morality, find steady employment, help society, use skills and judgment, try new methods, and feel a sense of accomplishment (Washington, 2019). Among master's- and doctorate-level psychologists working in correctional settings in North Carolina, the job characteristics that were associated with the highest satisfaction ratings included the following: autonomy; appropriate levels of responsibility; job security; relationships with coworkers, inmates, and supervisors; job success; personally meaningful work; and a sense of safety (MacKain et al., 2010). Safety, relationships with inmates, and salary were least associated with overall job satisfaction (MacKain et al., 2010).

APA DIVISIONS IN WASHINGTON (2019)

- 18 = Psychologists in Public Service
- 39 = Society for Psychoanalysis and Psychoanalytic Psychology
- 41 = American Psychology-Law Society
- 42 = Psychologists in Independent Practice

These studies paint a picture of a largely happy field of forensic mental health providers. However, the world has undergone significant shifts, including in the cost of education, cost of living, and overall stress and anxiety, much of which is associated with the observed trends in workplace attitude and behavior that we have noted. The world has changed dramatically in ways that have contributed to stress overall, as well as within the clinical field specifically, such as the COVID-19 pandemic, increased rates of mental health disorders, and ongoing national and global disasters and conflicts.

Psychology is a rewarding job as evidenced by research on the intrinsic value associated with this work. Despite being a rewarding job, a career as a psychologist also requires a lot of people. It can be emotionally exhausting, which may lead to vicarious trauma and compassion fatigue that in turn are associated with burnout and job turnover (Middleton & Potter, 2015). Forensic psychologists in particular may carry unique burdens related to the complex clinical cases of justice-involved individuals and the mountain to climb in support of systemic change within the justice system. As many areas of healthcare are becoming less resourced and more burdened, the supports that have proven so important may be harder to come by.

Although, as psychologists, we hope that you found this overview of research enlightening, the bottom line is that you are an n of 1. Your lived experience, ongoing circumstances, and individuality will dictate what job satisfaction and burnout as a forensic psychologist look like for you, and ultimately, whatever that experience ends up being will be more important than what the literature says. This is why it's important to check in with yourself along the way. Pivoting is always an option, and you may be surprised by the myriad ways in which you can meaningfully apply your forensic psychology background and expertise across a variety of contexts. But just like our hobbies and interests can wax and wane over time, so, too, can our job satisfaction. A lull in your career is not necessarily a sign that you should bolt. Maintaining professionalism, representing the field, and bolstering your reputation as a forensic psychologist will help you ride out those highs and lows regardless of where your career takes you and may ensure that the field is ready for you to return to should any career pivots end up showing you how much you loved the field to begin with.

CHAPTER TAKEAWAYS

Forensic psychology is a rich and diverse field, and numerous exciting career paths lay before you. Although we wish we could say with certainty that a job or organization exists out there that promises no bad days, this is not the reality we face. As you embark on your career, or potentially revisit the path you've already started down, bear in mind the importance of professionalism at every step of the way. And remember, our clinical training has prepared us well for the types of soft skills that can support you in representing yourself and the field well, regardless of workplace conflict and lulls in job satisfaction.

REFERENCES

American Psychological Association. (2013). Specialty guidelines for forensic psychology. *American Psychologist, 68*(1), 7–19. https://doi.org/10.1037/a0029889

American Psychological Association. (2017). *Ethical principles of psychologists and code of conduct.* https://www.apa.org/ethics/code/ethics-code-2017.pdf

Cote, C. (2023, September). 5 strategies for conflict resolution in the workplace. *Harvard Business School Online.* https://online.hbs.edu/blog/post/strategies-for-conflict-resolution-in-the-workplace

DeMatteo, D., Krauss, D. A., Fishel, S., & Wiltsie, K. (in press). *Forensic mental health practice and the law: A primer for clinicians, researchers, and consultants.* Oxford University Press.

Jackson, S. (2023, June). Top 10 workplace trends on TikTok this year: Quiet quitting, bare minimum Mondays, and more. *Business Insider: Careers.* https://www.businessinsider.com/top-work-trends-tiktok-quiet-quitting-hiring-act-your-wage-2023-5#10-shift-shock-14900-views-1

Jolaoso, C., & Main, K. (2023, May). 10 tips for effective communication in the workplace. *Forbes Advisor.* https://www.forbes.com/advisor/business/effective-communication-workplace/

Linehan, M. M. (2015). *DBT® Skills Training Manual* (2nd ed.). The Guilford Press.

MacKain, S. J., Myers, B., Ostapiej, L., & Newman, R. A. (2010). Job satisfaction among psychologists working in state prisons: The relative impact of facets assessing economics, management, relationships, and perceived organizational support. *Criminal Justice and Behavior, 37*(3), 306–318. https://doi.org/10.1177/0093854809357420

Middleton, J. S., & Potter, C. C. (2015). Relationship between vicarious traumatization and turnover among child welfare professionals. *Journal of Public Child Welfare, 9*, 195–216. https://doi.org/10.1080/15548732.2015.1021987

Novotney, A. (2022). Leaving academia: Psychologist who have made the jump from working in academic to industry or practice share their tips for how to use your PhD in other fields. *Monitor on Psychology, 53*(2). https://www.apa.org/monitor/2022/03/career-leaving-academia#:~:text=Many%20psychologists%20like%20Osborn%20say,impact%20on%20several%20different%20populations

Oore, G. D., Leiter, M. P., & LeBlanc, D. E. (2015). Individual and organizational factors promoting successful responses to workplace conflict. *Canadian Psychology, 56*(3), 301–310. https://doi.org/10.1037/cap0000032

Parker, K., & Horowitz, J. M. (2022, March). Majority of workers who quit a job in 2021 cite low pay, no opportunities for advancement, feeling disrespected. *Pew Research Center.* https://www.pewresearch.org/short-reads/2022/03/09/majority-of-workers-who-quit-a-job-in-2021-cite-low-pay-no-opportunities-for-advancement-feeling-disrespected/

Rupert, P. A., Miller, A. O., Tuminello Hartman, E. R., & Bryant, F. B. (2012). Predictors of career satisfaction among practicing psychologists. *Professional Psychology: Research and Practice, 43*(5), 495–502. https://doi.org/10.1037/a0029420

Washington, D. (2019). *Learning models, personality traits, and job satisfaction in forensic psychology practitioners* (Publication no. 7771) [Doctoral dissertation, Walden University.] Walden Dissertations and Doctoral Studies.

Yanchus, N. J., Periard, D., Moore, S. C., Carle, A. C., & Osatuke, K. (2015). Predictors of job satisfaction and turnover intention in VHA mental health employees: A comparison between psychiatrists, psychologists, social workers, and mental health nurses. *Human Service Organizations: Management, Leadership & Governance, 39*(3). https://doi.org/10.1080/23303131.2015.1014953

Index

For Product Safety Concerns and Information please contact our EU
representative GPSR@taylorandfrancis.com
Taylor & Francis Verlag GmbH, Kaufingerstraße 24, 80331 München, Germany